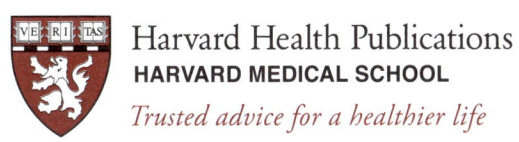 

Dear Reader,

Joint pain throbs, aches, and hurts. Quite likely, it makes you think twice about everyday tasks and pleasures like going for a brisk walk, lifting your grandchild or some grocery bags, chasing a tennis ball across the court, or driving a golf ball down the fairway. Sharp reminders of your limitations arrive thick and fast, practically every time you move.

Very often, the culprits behind joint pain are osteoarthritis, old injuries, repetitive or overly forceful movements during sports or work, posture problems, aging, or inactivity. Ignoring the pain won't make it go away. Nor will avoiding all motions that spark discomfort. In fact, limiting your movements can weaken muscles, compounding joint trouble, and affect your posture, setting off a cascade of further problems. And while pain relievers and cold or hot packs may offer quick relief, fixes like these are merely temporary.

By contrast, the right set of exercises can be a long-lasting way to tame ankle, knee, hip, or shoulder pain. Practiced regularly, the workouts in this report might permit you to postpone—or even avoid—surgery on a problem joint that has been worsening for years, by strengthening key supportive muscles and restoring flexibility. Over time, you may find limitations you've learned to work around will begin to ease. Tasks and opportunities for fun that you've weeded out of your repertoire by necessity may come back into reach, too.

Beyond the benefits to your joints, becoming more active can help you stay independent long into your later years. Regular activity is good for your heart and sharpens the mind. It nudges blood pressure down and morale up, eases stress, and shaves off unwanted pounds. Perhaps most importantly, it lessens your risk of dying prematurely. All of this can be achieved at a comfortable pace and very low cost in money or time—in fact, this report will show you how to fold many activities into your daily routine.

So select the specific workout you need. Check our safety tips, and then get started. We've combined our expertise in physical medicine and rehabilitation as well as personal training to prescribe gentle, effective warm-ups, stretches, and strengthening moves that will help you regain flexibility and build up supportive muscles. For avid golf and tennis players, or office athletes wincing from work-related repetitive motions, we've written a special section on wrists and elbows to get you back in the game.

Sincerely,

Edward M. Phillips, M.D.
Medical Editor

Josie Gardiner
Master Trainer

Joy Prouty
Master Trainer

Harvard Health Publications | Harvard Medical School | 10 Shattuck Street, Second Floor | Boston, MA 02115

Taking the first steps

Maybe you love to exercise. Or maybe you don't. Either way, we can show you how to set a course toward a healthier life by finding new ways to stay active. In this section, you'll find the answers to two very important questions: How much exercise should you aim for if you wish to stay healthy and independent? And, why bother to exercise at all?

How much exercise should you aim for?

The U.S. Department of Health and Human Services physical guidelines urge all adults—including people with various disabilities—to accumulate a weekly total of 150 minutes or more of moderate aerobic activity, or 75 minutes or more of vigorous activity, or an

Why bother to exercise?

Why should you exercise, particularly if it prompts twinges or outright pain in your joints? Put simply, staying active helps you feel, think, and look better. Regular exercise can take a load off aching joints by strengthening muscles and chiseling away excess pounds while easing swelling and pain. It allows some people to cut back on medications they take, such as drugs for high blood pressure or diabetes. And that can ease unwelcome side effects and save money.

Strong evidence from thousands of studies shows that engaging in regular exercise

- tacks years onto your life
- lowers your risks for early death, heart disease, stroke, type 2 diabetes, high blood pressure, high cholesterol, and metabolic syndrome (a complex problem that increases the risk for stroke, doubles risk for heart disease, and quintuples risk for diabetes by blending three or more of the following factors: high blood pressure, high triglycerides, low HDL cholesterol, a large waistline, and difficulty regulating blood sugar)
- helps keep your heart healthy by striking a better balance of blood lipids (HDL, LDL, and triglycerides), which prevents plaque buildup; helping arteries stay resilient despite aging; bumping up the number of blood vessels feeding the heart; reducing inflammation; and discouraging the formation of blood clots that can block coronary arteries
- lessens the likelihood of getting colon and breast cancers
- helps keep you from gaining weight
- may help with weight loss (and maintaining weight loss) when combined with the proper diet, which in turn may help slow, or even reverse, knee problems
- strengthens muscles, lungs, and heart
- helps prevent falls that can lead to debilitating fractures and loss of independence
- eases depression
- boosts mental sharpness in older adults.

Emerging evidence suggests that regular exercise also

- improves functional abilities in older adults—that is, being able to walk up stairs or through a store, heft groceries, rise from a chair without help, and perform a multitude of other activities that permit independence or bring joy to our lives
- helps lessen abdominal obesity, which plays a role in many serious ailments, including heart disease, diabetes, and stroke
- boosts bone density (provided the exercises are weight-bearing, meaning that they work against gravity)
- lowers risk for hip fractures
- leads to better sleep
- lowers risks for lung and endometrial cancer.

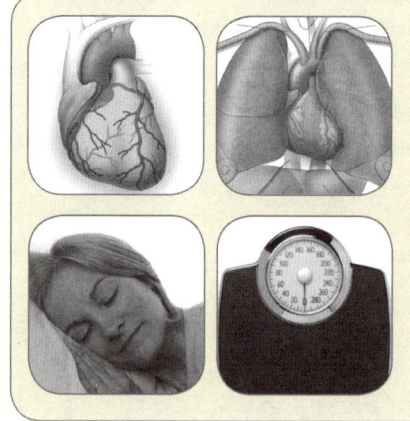

Regular exercise lowers your risk for heart disease, strengthens your heart and lungs, improves sleep, and helps you maintain a healthy weight or lose weight.

The Joint Pain Relief Workout

equivalent mix of the two, spread throughout the week. That's sufficient to gain all the health benefits described in "Why bother to exercise?" on page 2.

One way to attain this is engaging in 30 minutes of physical activity per day, five days a week, as the American College of Sports Medicine and the American Heart Association recommend in collaborative guidelines. Or you can tot up your weekly time in exercise sessions of various lengths throughout the week. Keep in mind:

- Ten minutes of vigorous activity equals approximately 20 minutes of moderate activity. (When doing moderate activity, you can talk, but not sing; during vigorous activity, you can say only a few words without pausing to breathe.)
- Activity should last at least 10 minutes at a time.
- Twice-weekly sessions of strength exercises focused on the legs, hips, back, abdomen, chest, shoulders, and arms are recommended, too.
- Balance exercises are suggested, as well, for older adults at risk of falling.

If you're ready for a challenge, doubling your weekly exercise time—300 minutes of moderate aerobic activity, or 150 minutes of vigorous activity—boosts health benefits.

What if you're shaking your head at the thought of doing this much activity? That's not unlikely, especially if joint pain has been slowing you down. If that's true for you, just remember that any amount of exercise beats none. Try to do as much as possible. Even short stints of activity (five minutes of walking several times a day to help you build endurance) are a good first step toward meeting a bigger goal.

Stop sitting

Even if you're reasonably active, hours of sitting—whether reading a book, working on the computer, or watching TV—tighten hip flexor muscles. Overly tight hip flexors affect gait and balance, making activities like walking harder and perhaps even setting you up for a fall. Plus, tight hip flexors may contribute to lower back pain, a scourge many people suffer with every day.

If that's not enough to get you moving, consider this: research shows that many people spend more than half their waking hours sitting down. And observational studies suggest habitual inactivity raises risks for obesity, diabetes, cardiovascular disease, deep-vein thrombosis, and metabolic syndrome.

Safety first

While it's tempting to flip right to the workout section on page 18, it's best think about safety first. The goal of this report is to ease pain and prevent injuries, not raise the odds of both. Start with the tips in this section aimed at helping you work out safely and effectively. Read the list of warning signs that should prompt you to call a doctor for advice, and check the simple equipment you'll need to do your workouts. Then, you'll be ready to get started.

First, it helps to understand how joints work. Joints are junctions in the body that link bones together. A joint's structure—whether a hinge, pivot, ball-in-socket, or other formation—allows movement in many directions. Inside the joint, cartilage cushions the intersections between bones and absorbs synovial fluid, a lubricant that helps protect bones from being worn away over time by friction. Ligaments made of strong, usually inelastic tissue bind and stabilize joints. Stretchy cords of tissue called tendons tether muscle to bone and cartilage. The brain coordinates the lightning-quick signals that pass along nerve pathways to contract and relax opposing muscles. The muscles attach to tendons, which tug on bones, allowing the body to walk and jump, dance and run—that is, to move in any way you choose.

Unfortunately, many of us choose to move less and less as the years pass by. And joint pain often provides a seemingly ironclad excuse to pare back activities. By letting joint pain sideline you, though, you squelch many joys in life. Still worse, you compromise your health, well-being, and independence. And often, inactivity actually makes joint pain escalate. This report encourages you to buck this dismal trend by pairing gentle, targeted joint workouts with a simple walking plan that could add years to your life while changing it for the better. Before getting started, though, you'll want to review the section below to see if you should discuss this exercise plan with your doctor.

Do you need to see a doctor?

Any doctor will tell you exercise is essential for a healthy life. But are the exercises we're recommending safe for you? Generally, light to moderate exercise is safe for healthy adults. Almost anyone—healthy or not—can safely take up walking. But before starting the workouts in this report, it's best to check with your doctor if

- you've been experiencing pain in joints, particularly if you aren't usually active
- you have a chronic or unstable health condition, such as heart disease or several risk factors for heart disease, asthma or another respiratory ailment, high blood pressure, osteoporosis, or diabetes.

You may want to use a helpful tool developed by the Canadian Society for Exercise Physiology. Called the Physical Activity Readiness Questionnaire (PAR-Q), this set of questions can help you determine whether you should talk to a doctor before embarking

> ### ▶ Warning signs
>
> Call a doctor for advice if you experience any of these warning signs during or after exercise:
>
> - sudden, sharp, or intense pain
> - pain lasting one or two weeks (as distinct from delayed-onset muscle soreness, a normal response to taxing your muscles that usually peaks 24 to 48 hours after a workout and gradually abates)
> - dizziness; faintness; chest pain, pressure, heaviness, or tightness; or significant or persistent shortness of breath
> - in hot, humid weather: headache, dizziness, nausea, faintness, cramps, or palpitations, which are the likely signs of overheating.

on or ramping up an exercise program. You can find it at www.health.harvard.edu/PAR-Q.

If you do need to speak to your doctor, ask if you can follow the program described in specific joint workouts in this report. If you're not currently exercising, discuss our proposed walking plan, too. Your doctor may feel these workouts are fine as long as you start gradually and build up slowly, or may want to modify the program to make it safer for you. If necessary, your doctor can refer you to a physiatrist, physical therapist, or another health care specialist like a cardiologist or rheumatologist for further evaluation. Occasionally, a doctor may recommend working out with the supervision of an experienced personal trainer or a health professional.

■ **Physiatrists,** also known as rehabilitation physicians, are board-certified medical doctors who specialize in treating nerve, muscle, and bone conditions that affect movement. Knee or shoulder injuries, debilitating arthritis or obesity, stroke, back problems, and repetitive stress injuries are a few examples. A physiatrist can tailor an exercise prescription to enhance recovery after surgery or an injury, or to help you work out with limitations posed by pain or limited movement. He or she can also tell you whether certain types of exercise will be helpful or harmful given your specific health history.

■ **Physical therapists** help restore abilities to people with health conditions or injuries affecting muscles, joints, bones, or nerves. Their expertise can be valuable if, for instance, you have suffered a lingering sprain or are recovering from a heart attack or hip replacement. Some specialize in cardiopulmonary rehabilitation, orthopedics, sports medicine, geriatrics, or other areas. Physical therapists must graduate from an accredited physical therapy program, which they enter after receiving a bachelor's degree; most accredited physical therapy programs in the United States offer doctoral degrees. In addition, they must pass a national exam given by the Federation of State Boards of Physical Therapy and be licensed by their state. Specialists complete advanced training and additional national exams to become board certified.

■ **Physical therapy assistants** provide physical therapy services under the supervision of a physical

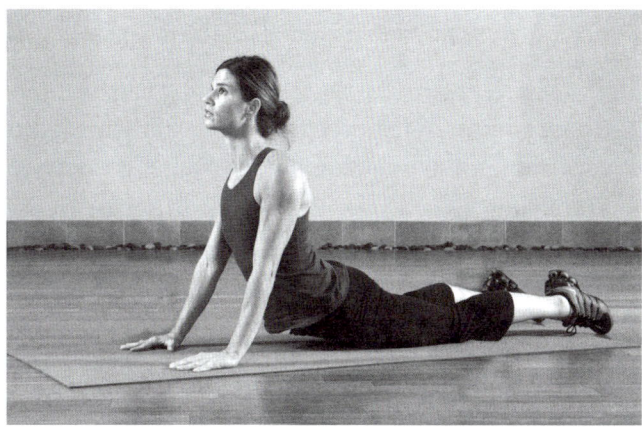

Although there isn't much scientific evidence favoring a cool-down following a light to moderate workout, the end of your session is an excellent time to stretch since your muscles are well warmed up.

therapist; they must complete a two-year associate's degree, pass a national exam, and, in most states, be licensed.

■ **Personal trainers** are fitness specialists who can help ensure that you're doing exercises properly. While encouraging and motivating you, they can teach new skills, fine-tune your form, change up routines to beat boredom, and safely push you to the next level. No nationwide licensing requirements exist for personal trainers, although standards for the accrediting fitness organizations that train them have been set by the National Commission for Certifying Agencies. Two well-respected organizations that offer programs of study for personal trainers are the American College of Sports Medicine (ACSM) and the American Council on Exercise (ACE); others include the National Council on Strength and Fitness (NCSF), the National Strength and Conditioning Association (NSCA), and the National Academy of Sports Medicine (NASM). All fitness organizations have different requirements for training and expertise. Some trainers specialize in working with particular populations—for example, older adults or athletes—and may have taken courses and possibly certifying exams in these areas.

Six all-around exercise tips

Whatever kind of exercise you choose to do, following these general tips can help you protect yourself from injury and illness.

1. **Warm up properly.** Allot several minutes for this before a workout.
2. **Boost your activity level gradually over time.** Start slowly, building up gradually over time. If you stop exercising for a while, drop back if necessary by doing fewer repetitions or sets, then build back up.
3. **Pay attention to your body.** Don't exercise when you're sick or feeling overly fatigued. Fatigue often leads to injuries.
4. **Avoid overtraining.** Follow the guidelines for how often to do exercises. Training too hard or too often can cause overuse injuries like stress fractures, stiff or sore joints and muscles, and inflamed tendons and ligaments.
5. **Respect the weather.** When humidity is high or the thermometer is expected to reach 80° F, exercise during cooler morning or evening hours or in an air-conditioned space. When exercising outside in cold weather, dress in layers, including gloves and hat. If you have asthma or other respiratory problems, plan to exercise indoors when air quality is especially unhealthy. Seasonal allergy sufferers benefit from this, too, when pollen counts are high or other allergens abound.
6. **Stay hydrated.** Drink sufficient fluids throughout the day and while exercising, especially if it's hot or humid.

Five strength training tips

When doing strength training, including the workouts in this report, follow these tips to help prevent injury.

1. **Use light weight or resistance only.** Strength is built by working a muscle against resistance. (Exercise programs that do this are called strength training, resistance training, or weight training programs.) The resistance can be supplied by a hand weight like a dumbbell; elastic resistance bands or tubing; a weight machine; or your own body weight, as push-ups neatly illustrate. All of the workouts in this report emphasize building up muscle strength very slowly. When an exercise calls for hand weights, use no more than 1 to 3 pounds. When using resistance bands and tubing, select light to medium resistance.
2. **Focus on form.** Good form means aligning your body as described in exercise instructions and moving smoothly through an exercise. Holding your body in a specific position while consciously contracting and releasing certain muscles allows you to isolate a muscle group. Poor form can slow gains and trigger injuries.
3. **Tempo, tempo.** Work evenly at the tempo specified in each exercise. Control is very important. Counting off the tempo aloud helps you stay in control, which enhances gains and helps you avoid injuries. It also ensures that you're breathing, rather than holding your breath.
4. **Breathe.** Blood pressure rises if you hold your breath during resistance exercises. Exhale as you work against gravity by lifting, pushing, or pulling; inhale as you release. During warm-ups and stretches, breathe comfortably.
5. **Give muscles time off.** Strength training causes tiny tears in muscle tissue. Muscles grow stronger as the tears knit up. Allow at least 48 hours between strength training sessions on a particular group of muscles to allow them to recover.

Four stretching tips

Using proper technique for stretching can protect your muscles and joints.

1. **Warm up first.** Much like taffy, muscles stretch more easily when warm. Doing the warm-ups for each workout or taking a warm shower or bath will do the trick.
2. **Feel no pain.** Stretch only to the point of mild tension, never to the point of pain. If a stretch hurts, stop immediately! Reset your position carefully and try again. With time and practice, your flexibility will improve.
3. **Breathe.** Breathe comfortably when stretching.
4. **Practice often.** You'll see the best gains if you stretch frequently—several times a day on as many days of the week as possible.

Posture, alignment, and angles: Striking the right pose

Posture counts when you're exercising. Aligning your body properly is the key to good form, which results in greater gains and fewer injuries. Few people have perfect posture, so we recommend quick posture checks before and during each exercise. If possible, look in a mirror as you do each exercise.

When an exercise in our workouts calls for you to stand up straight, that means

- chin parallel to the floor
- both shoulders even (roll them up, back, and down to help achieve this)
- both arms at your sides with elbows straight and even
- abdominal muscles pulled in
- both hips even
- both knees even and pointing straight ahead
- both feet pointing straight ahead
- body weight distributed evenly on both feet.

> Do quick posture checks before and during each exercise.

Whether you're standing or seated, neutral posture requires you to keep your chin parallel to the floor; your shoulders, hips, and knees at even heights; and your knees and feet pointing straight ahead. A neutral spine takes into account the slight natural curves of the spine—don't flex it or arch it to overemphasize the curve of the lower back. A neutral wrist is firm and straight, not bent upward or downward. And neutral alignment means keeping your body in a straight line from head to toe except for the slight natural curves of the spine.

When angles appear in exercise instructions, try visualizing a 90-degree angle as an L or two adjacent sides of a square. To visualize a 30-degree angle, mentally slice the 90-degree angle into thirds, or picture the distance between the hands of a clock at one o'clock.

▶ Hip bone connected to the leg bone

The old song "Dry Bones" had it right. The toe bone is connected to the foot bone, and the foot bone is connected to the ankle bone, and so on up the long, linked chain of bones that make up a complete skeleton. So, for example, injuring your left ankle completely alters your gait. To take the weight off the painful foot, you move more quickly than usual on your left side, lurching forward repeatedly onto your right leg. This potent combination of force and misalignment can trigger bursitis and pain in your right hip. Thus, new problems may zigzag up the body, making you vulnerable to further injuries, particularly if muscles supporting other joints are weak. If your body stages a general slowdown in response to all the new discomforts, other muscles eventually become deconditioned, too.

Take steps to minimize misalignments, when possible. Be aware of pain and restrictions in range of motion as you increase your physical activity. Pause occasionally to take stock of your body position and actively practice good posture. Wear supportive shoes (and orthotics to align your feet properly if your doctor feels you need them). Choose bags that distribute weight evenly, such as backpacks.

Equipment: Choosing the right stuff

We designed our workouts for home or gym. Look at the start of each workout description to see what equipment you'll need; each workout uses some, not all, of the equipment listed below. When equipment is listed as optional, you'll need it if you choose to do a harder or easier variation of certain exercises. Below are some buying tips for each of the items mentioned in our workouts.

■ **Ankle weights.** These are used to increase resistance in the harder variations of certain exercises. Choose padded, adjustable ankle weights with 1-pound bars so you can vary the weight as needed.

■ **Chair.** Choose a sturdy chair that won't tip over easily. A plain wooden dining chair without arms or heavy padding works well.

■ **Hand weights.** Our joint workouts use very light weights of 1 to 3 pounds, or occasionally 3 to 5 pounds. D-shaped weights and padded weights are easier to hold. Kits that let you screw weights onto a central bar save storage space.

■ **Hand towel.** A small hand towel tucked under your elbow anchors your upper arm during a few exercises. This helps isolate the muscles that the exercise is designed to strengthen. Any hand towel will do.

■ **Mat.** Choose a well-padded, nonslip mat for floor exercises. Yoga mats are readily available. A thick carpet or towels will do in a pinch.

■ **Resistance bands.** These wide, stretchy strips are available in several levels of resistance, designated by different colors and ranging from very light to very heavy. Resistance bands are often used for rehabilitation exercises after injuries or surgery. The strips can be knotted into a loop when an exercise requires this (see "Point and flex," page 21), or tied securely around a column, banister, or doorknob. Choose light- to medium-resistance bands in 6-foot lengths (or cut rolls of bands to this length yourself).

■ **Resistance tubing.** Look for tubing in several levels of resistance and with padded handles on the ends. Different colors designate varying amounts of resistance from very light to very heavy. For these workouts, choose light to medium resistance. Also look for a brand with a door attachment, which allows you to anchor the tubing in place when doing certain exercises.

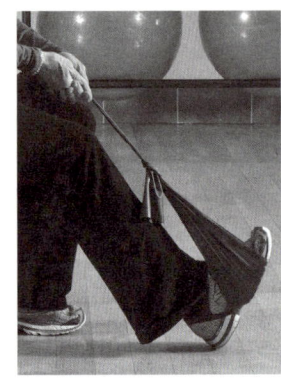

Before each use, make sure the band has no nicks or cuts that will cause it to break. For safety, replace resistance bands often.

■ **Rubber ball.** Choose a ball you can comfortably fit in your hand. The squishier the ball, the easier the workout, so select a firmer rubber ball when you're ready for more of a challenge.

■ **Shoes.** Choosing the right shoe for the task—running, walking, tennis, golf—is important. Running or walking shoes lose cushioning and support over time, so be sure to replace them regularly. Some experts suggest buying new ones every 350 to 550 miles.

■ **Stability ball.** Stability balls come in several sizes (55 cm, 65 cm, and 75 cm are most common, but smaller and larger balls are available). To select a ball, check the package for a size chart based on your height. When you sit on a ball, your hips and knees should both be at 90-degree angles. Select a durable, high-quality ball, such as Max Fitness or Spri brands.

■ **Yoga strap.** This is a nonelastic cotton or nylon strap of 6 feet or longer that helps you position your body properly while doing certain stretches. Choose a strap with a D-ring or buckle fastener on one end. This allows you to put a loop around a foot or leg and then grasp the other end of the strap. ▼

Getting started

Often, the slide toward an increasingly sedentary life starts with painful joints because discomfort curtails activities. Although a doctor may prescribe temporary rest after an injury or surgery, week after week of inactivity compromises your health and abilities. Our simple walking plan can help you turn around this unhealthy trend. If walking isn't possible, see "When walks are too hard" on page 10 for alternative activities.

A simple cardio workout

Like all aerobic (cardio) activities, walking tunes up the heart and lungs while burning calories. Because it doesn't jar joints terribly or raise the heart rate to dangerous levels, it's safe for almost everyone. Our walking plan ramps up slowly. Follow these tips to get the most from your walks:

■ **Find safe places to walk.** Quiet streets with sidewalks, park trails, athletic tracks at local schools, or indoor malls are safest. If you're looking for a flat surface, the latter two choices are best.

■ **Buy a good pair of shoes.** Look for thick, flexible soles that cushion your feet and elevate your heel a half to three-quarters of an inch above the sole. Choose shoes with "breathable" uppers, such as nylon mesh or leather.

■ **Dress for comfort and safety.** Since exercise warms your body, wear lighter clothes than you'd need if standing still. Dress in layers so you can peel off garments if you get hot. Wear a hat with a brim and sunblock when needed. Light-colored clothes and reflective strips, a reflective vest, or a lightweight flashing light can help drivers notice you.

■ **Do a warm-up.** Walk at a slower pace for several minutes as you start out.

■ **Practice good technique.** For example:
- Walk at a steady, moderate-intensity pace (see Table 2 or "A walking plan," below). Slow down if you're too breathless to carry on a conversation.

▶ A walking plan

Our walking plan is designed to safely boost your physical activity even if you are very sedentary. It's the minutes that count, not the miles. If you aren't in the habit of exercising, start at the beginning. If you're already exercising, start at the level that best matches your current routine and build from there. You may advance more slowly by repeating a level for an additional week. Or, if the plan is too easy, you may add walking time more quickly. Once you're in shape, feel free to change time and days while still aiming for at least 150 minutes of walking per week.

Looking for more of a challenge? Add time, distance, or hills to improve endurance. If walking is difficult, see "When walks are too hard," page 10.

Remember:
- Begin your walk at a slower pace for several minutes to warm up. After your walk is an excellent time to stretch warmed muscles.
- A brisk (moderate) pace makes singing difficult, but you should be able to talk (see Table 2 on page 15).
- If you like, you can divide daily walking time into 10-minute chunks (three chunks equals 30 minutes).

Week	Sessions per week	Daily minutes of brisk walking	Total weekly minutes
Week 1	2	5	10
Week 2	3	5	15
Week 3	4	5	20
Week 4	5	5	25
Week 5	5	10	50
Week 6	5	20	100
Week 7	5	25	125
Week 8	5	30	150

One way to measure walking speed is to count steps per minute with a watch and pedometer. A moderate (brisk) walking speed is a safe goal for most people. Provided you're walking on level ground, you can use the following as general guidance to gauge your pace:

Slow = 80 steps per minute
Moderate (brisk) = 100 steps per minute
Fast = 120 steps per minute
Race walking = More than 120 steps per minute

- Keep your head up and back straight. Lift your chest and shoulders. Gently contract your stomach muscles.

- Keeping toes pointed straight ahead, land on your heel, then roll forward onto the ball of your foot and push off from your toes. Walking flat-footed or only on the ball of your foot may lead to soreness and fatigue. Take long, easy strides, letting your arms swing loosely at your sides.

- If you want to boost your speed, bend your elbows at a 90-degree angle and swing your hands from waist to chest height. Take quicker steps, not longer ones.

- When walking faster or going up hills, lean forward slightly.

Stretch after walking. Stretching when your muscles are warm improves your range of motion.

When walks are too hard

Strengthening muscles that support weak hip, knee, or ankle joints and working on flexibility can help you return to walking comfortably. But if these trouble spots make our walking plan too hard for you right now, try some of these other options:

- elliptical trainer
- hand-crank bike
- kayaking simulator
- recumbent or upright stationary bike
- recumbent or upright stepper
- rowing machine
- swimming
- tai chi
- water aerobics
- water walking.

By working large muscles, which bumps up your heart rate and breathing to circulate oxygen more quickly throughout your body, all of these choices enhance cardiovascular fitness as well as walking does, while going easy on the joints. Some equipment—like elliptical trainers, kayaking simulators, and recumbent stationary bikes—is available at gyms and exercise rehabilitation centers.

Yoga is less likely to supply cardiovascular benefits. Still, it's an excellent form of exercise that strengthens muscles and increases flexibility.

Why weight matters

Being overweight raises your risk for developing osteoarthritis in a weight-

Table 1 Normal, overweight, or obese?

The body mass index (BMI) is an index of weight by height. The definitions of normal, overweight, and obese were established after researchers examined the BMIs of millions of people and correlated them with rates of illness and death. These studies identified the normal BMI range as that associated with the lowest rates of illness and death. Obesity has been further subdivided into three classes. People may be candidates for weight-loss surgery if they have class III obesity, or if they have class II obesity and diabetes or another serious, weight-related medical condition.

HEIGHT	BODY WEIGHT IN POUNDS				
4'10"	89–119	120–143	144–167	168–191	192+
4'11"	92–124	125–148	149–173	174–198	199+
5'0"	95–128	129–153	154–179	179–204	205+
5'1"	98–132	133–158	159–185	186–211	212+
5'2"	101–136	137–164	165–191	192–218	219+
5'3"	105–141	142–169	170–197	198–225	226+
5'4"	108–145	146–174	175–204	205–232	233+
5'5"	111–150	151–180	181–210	211–240	241+
5'6"	115–155	156–186	187–216	217–247	248+
5'7"	118–159	160–191	192–223	224–255	256+
5'8"	122–164	165–197	198–230	231–262	263+
5'9"	126–169	170–203	204–236	237–270	271+
5'10"	129–174	175–209	210–243	244–278	279+
5'11"	133–179	180–215	216–250	251–286	287+
6'0"	137–184	185–221	222–258	259–294	295+
6'1"	140–189	190–227	228–265	266–302	303+
6'2"	145–194	195–233	234–272	273–311	312+
6'3"	149–200	201–240	241–279	279–319	320+
6'4"	153–205	206–246	247–287	288–328	329+
BMI	18.5–24.9	25–29.9	30–34.9	35–39.9	40+
	NORMAL	OVER-WEIGHT	CLASS I OBESITY	CLASS II OBESITY	CLASS III OBESITY

bearing joint like the knee—and even in the hand, according to some research, since inflammatory factors related to weight might exacerbate this condition. Simply walking across level ground puts up to one-and-a-half times your body weight on your knees. That means a 200-pound man will deliver 300 pounds of pressure to his knee with each step. Off level ground, the news is worse: each knee bears two to three times your body weight when you go up and down stairs, and four to five times your body weight when you squat to tie a shoelace or pick up an item you dropped.

Fortunately, strengthening your quadriceps (the muscles on the fronts of the thighs) changes the equation, and so does losing weight. Each pound you lose reduces knee pressure in every step you take. One study found that the risk of developing osteoarthritis dropped 50% with each 11-pound weight loss among younger obese women. If older men lost enough weight to shift from an obese classification to just overweight—that is, from a body mass index (BMI) of 30 or higher down to one that fell between 25 and 29.9—the researchers estimated knee osteoarthritis would decrease by a fifth. For older women, that shift would cut knee osteoarthritis by a third.

To find your BMI, see Table 1.

The best tactics for losing weight

Aerobic activity, such as walking or an alternative (see "When walks are too hard," page 10), is best for aiding in weight loss and helping you maintain a healthy weight. But by itself, stepping up activity is rarely enough to help you lose weight (see "Why it's tough to lose weight with activity alone," below). Every pound you'd like to shed represents roughly 3,500 calories. So, if you're hoping to lose half a pound to one pound a week, you need to knock off 250 to 500 calories a day. Vaporizing half through exercising and half by cutting calories from your diet is a good mix. Aiming at the lower number—125 calories shed through exercise and 125 calories shaved off your diet—can help ensure success.

It's wise to keep in mind that the math works in the other direction, too: if you don't burn a single calorie through exercise and you add 250 calories a day through more nibbling, you'd rack up an extra 26 pounds a year. Indulging in an extra 100 calories a day without burning them off packs 10 pounds a year onto you. Over time, daily indulgences like a scoop or two of ice cream, an energy bar, or a raid on the cookie or candy jar can tip the scales against us.

What sort of diet is best? Try to stick with diets that emphasize healthy choices: lots of fruits, vegetables, and whole grains; fish, lean poultry, beans, and legumes as protein sources; healthful oils; and a sprinkling of nuts.

Why it's tough to lose weight with activity alone

By rights, pounds ought to peel off as your activity level rises. Alas, it rarely works this way, for these reasons among others:

Virtue is rarely its own reward. Ever treat yourself to a cookie or an extra dollop of dinner on a day when you walked or worked out? It's a common impulse that undermines people. Usually, we burn far fewer calories than we think through exercise. It's incredibly easy to replace what you burn: 20 minutes of brisk walking burns 69 calories for a 120-pound person; 86 calories for a 150-pound person; and 103 calories for a 180-pound person. But a small cookie can cost you 50 to 60 calories, a serving of chips tallies 150 calories, and a half cup of ice cream can be 140 calories (and many of us scoop more than that into our bowls). Healthier rewards range from appreciating the effects of exercise—feeling more energetic, calmer, or stronger, for example—to planning a night out or promising yourself new exercise gear or a new CD if you stick with your program.

The calorie counter is not set at zero. Let's say you loll around in bed day and night for a 24-hour span. You'd be burning calories at a low, steady speed known as your basal metabolic rate (BMR). Activity temporarily bumps up the number of calories burned; then the needle falls back to your BMR if you settle back into your pillows. While it's true that 20 minutes of brisk walking burns 69 calories for our 120-pound subject, you'd need to subtract basal metabolic rate to get a true count of calories burned just through adding walking. If you're curious, run your vital stats through the basal metabolic rate calculator and the activity calculator on the Discovery Health website. (Find them quickly at www.health.harvard.edu/basal and www.health.harvard.edu/activitycalc.) Remember to divide by 24 to get your hourly BMR. And divide that again if you're interested in smaller increments of time.

Usually, we burn far fewer calories than we think through exercise.

Dig deep for motivation

Need more motivation to make a start or stick to it? Welcome to the club. Often, the hardest part of a workout is digging up the motivation to do it. While exercise is great medicine, it only works if you carve out time to do it regularly. Here are a few tips:

■ **Find the time.** Skip several half-hour TV shows a week or work out while watching. Get up half an hour earlier each day for a morning workout. If big blocks of time aren't falling into your lap, break it up. Try 10-minute walks, or half a workout in the morning and half in the evening.

■ **Build active moments into your day.** Start small and build up by choosing among options like these: Take stairs, not elevators. When commuting, get off the bus or subway a stop or two ahead, or park farther away from your workplace. While on the phone, try a few stretches, pace, or do simple exercises like lunges, squats, and heel raises. Bike or walk to work.

My monthly log: Planning your workouts and walking program

WEEK	MONDAY	TUESDAY	WEDNESDAY
Example	Ankles: Full workout 7:30–8:00 p.m. Walking 12:30–12:50 p.m.	Walking 12:30–12:50 p.m.	Ankles: Full workout 7:30–8:00 p.m.
1			
2			
3			
4			
5			

When running errands within a reasonable radius, park your car in one spot and walk to different shops. Replace your desk and desk chair with a standing desk. Try substituting a stability ball for your desk chair a few hours a day. Rake leaves and shovel snow instead of using a leaf blower or snowblower.

Find a workout buddy. Workouts with a friend are more fun, plus you're less likely to cancel on the spur of the moment.

Brainstorm solutions. Understanding likely bumps in the road and planning solutions can help keep you on track.

- Need the okay to start exercising? Call your doctor today. It may help to fax or send a copy of the workout and walking plan, then follow up with a phone call to discuss it.

- Bugged by bad weather or early darkness? Buy equipment necessary for exercising at home, join a gym, try a class in your community, or walk the mall or an indoor athletic track at a local school.

- Feeling sick? Take time off to recover, then start at an easier-than-usual pace and work back up.

- Boredom? Join a class, change up your exercise routine, or find a workout buddy.

- Just don't feel motivated? Remind yourself of your goals, plan small rewards, ask a friend to check up on you, or consider working out with a personal trainer.

Now it's your turn. Fill out the planning worksheet below, brainstorming solutions as you go.

Month: _____

THURSDAY	FRIDAY	SATURDAY	SUNDAY
Walking *12:30–12:50 p.m.*	*Walking* *12:30–12:50 p.m.*	*Walking* *12:30–12:50 p.m.*	

Planning worksheet

Filling in this worksheet will help you set goals and jump hurdles. Start by listing what you stand to gain. This could be the extra push you need to stay on track. Also note how active you are now, so you'll know if you're getting sufficient exercise to stay healthy and independent (see "How much exercise should you aim for?" on page 2).

Make a copy of the worksheet. Write down your answers, and then fill in the monthly log. Tack it up on your refrigerator or another spot where you'll see it every day. Share your goals with family and friends, so that they can encourage you, too.

1. What will I gain?

Is your shoulder keeping you away from tennis or making it hard to lift a child, grandchild, or bag of groceries? Has your knee put the kibosh on walking, hikes, running, or just climbing stairs comfortably? Think about what you're missing out on, what you need to be able to do, and what you might enjoy trying.

_____

_____

_____

My first goal is to:

❏ Build up my ankles so I can _____.

❏ Build up my knees so I can _____.

❏ Build up my shoulders so I can _____.

❏ Build up my hips so I can _____.

❏ Build up my wrists and elbows so I can_____.

My additional goals are to:

❏ enhance my overall health

❏ tone my muscles

❏ extend my endurance

❏ improve my balance

❏ lose _____ pounds in the next _____ weeks for the benefit of my knees and all-around health. (Work toward an initial goal of losing 5% to 10% of your weight by losing half a pound to one pound a week. If you weigh 200 pounds, that's 10 to 20 pounds.)

I'd like to:

❏ do the ankle workout

❏ do the knee workout

❏ do the hip workout

❏ do the shoulder workout

❏ do the wrist and elbow workout

❏ add the walking program or another cardio workout to enhance my overall health and improve my endurance.

2. How can I make it over the hurdles?

What might keep you from exercising regularly? When you run into hurdles—boredom, time crunches, and other common setbacks—reminding yourself of the pledges below can help you make it over them. It pays to think ahead about what might derail you, then brainstorm solutions that will help you stick with your plan. Here are some solutions for common problems.

❏ I will stay excited by rotating activities and trying out new sports, interactive computer games like Wii Fit, dancing, or other enjoyable activities.

❏ I will plan ahead for short winter days and tough weather conditions (too hot, too cold, too icy, too rainy, too humid) by finding indoor spaces for my workouts, such as a gym, local community center, mall, or my home.

❏ If I find it hard to exercise at the end of a long day, I'll choose times of day when I feel more energetic.

❏ I will make small promises I can keep, allowing me to celebrate successes and make slow, steady gains.

❏ I will make a game out of finding as many ways as possible to slip exercise into my day through simple steps like taking the stairs, walking the dog, parking in one spot to run several errands, marching or jogging in place during TV commercials, or fitting in a few stretches or exercises before meals, during breaks, or even while on the phone.

❏ I will invite friends, family, or co-workers to join me for walks, sports, and interactive computer games like Wii Fit—and possibly even match me in friendly competition (biggest exerciser, anyone?).

What else might help me stick to my plan?

_____

_____

My plan:

Make copies of the monthly log, then jot down the title of the workout you'll do, penciling in the time slot and day you've chosen. Remember the advice to start slow and build gradually. Pencil in your walking program, too, by adding time and days from "A walking plan" on page 9. Then check off every workout you complete. Asking a friend to hold you accountable—or striking a similar bargain with your doctor—may encourage you to exercise. If so, copy the completed log and send it to your friend or doctor at the end of each month.

Using the workouts

This section explains terms used in the workouts and answers six common questions. Table 2 describes cues to help you measure the intensity of various activities, including walking.

What information is in each workout?

When you turn to the workout you've chosen—for instance, shoulders or knees—you'll find each exercise has certain specific information and instructions, as explained in this section.

■ **Repetitions (or reps).** Each rep is a single complete exercise. It's fine if you can't do all the reps at first. Focus on quality—good form comes first—rather than quantity. Gradually increase reps as you improve.

■ **Sets.** One set is a specific number of repetitions. In our workouts, 10 reps typically add up to a single set. Usually, we suggest doing one to three sets.

■ **Intensity.** Intensity measures how hard you work during an exercise. Pay attention to objective physiological cues like breathing, talking, and sweating, or you can measure intensity subjectively through perceived exertion (see Table 2).

■ **Tempo.** This provides the count for the key movements in an exercise. A 3-1-3 tempo requires you to count to three as you lower a weight, pause for one beat, then count to three as you lift the weight. Here's how tempo works during the movements in "Wall push-up with stability ball" (see page 37): Slowly count 1-2-3 while bending your elbows to lower your upper body toward the wall. Pause for one second. Then count 3-2-1 as you return to the starting position. To avoid hurrying, it helps to count while watching or listening to seconds tick by on a clock. When you can no longer maintain the recommended tempo, stop that particular exercise even if you haven't finished all of the reps.

■ **Hold.** Hold tells you the number of seconds to pause while holding a pose during an exercise. You'll see this in stretches, which are held 10 to 30 seconds. While starting out at 10 seconds is fine, gradually extending that until you can comfortably hold the stretch for 30 seconds will give you better results. So, too, will practicing flexibility exercises every day rather than just a few times a week.

■ **Rest.** Resting gives your muscles a chance to recharge, which helps you maintain good form. No rest is needed during warm-ups or after stretches unless otherwise specified.

■ **Starting position.** This describes how to position your body before starting the exercise.

■ **Movement.** Here you'll find out how to perform one complete repetition correctly.

■ **Tips and techniques.** We offer two or three pointers to help you maintain good form and make the greatest gains from the exercise.

■ **Too hard?** This section gives you an option for making the exercise easier.

■ **Too easy?** This section gives you an option for making the exercise more challenging.

Table 2 How hard am I working?

INTENSITY	IT FEELS…	YOU ARE…
Light	Easy	Breathing easily Warming up, but not yet sweating Able to talk—or even sing an aria if you have the talent
Light to moderate	You're working, but not too hard	Breathing easily Sweating lightly Still finding it easy to talk or sing
Moderate	You're working	Breathing faster Starting to sweat more Able to talk, not able to sing
Moderate to high	You're really working	Huffing and puffing Sweating Able to talk in short sentences, but concentrating more on exercise than conversation
High	You're working very hard, almost out of gas	Breathing hard Sweating hard Finding talking difficult

Answers to six common questions

If you haven't been working out regularly, or even if you have, you may have some questions about getting started on the workouts in this report. Here we answer some common questions.

1. Which workout should I do?

That depends on which joints are bothering you. If it's an ankle, turn to "Ankle workout" (see page 18); if it's your hips, turn to "Hip workout" (see page 30). What if it's both? It's safe to do both routines as long as the problems you're experiencing are described in the workout introductions. If you have more significant joint problems, or if you have any doubts, see your doctor before you start any workout!

Pair the workout or workouts you choose with the weekly walking program or another choice (see "When walks are too hard," page 10) to get the cardio tune-up your body needs.

2. What if I can't do all the reps or sets suggested?

Quality is much more important than quantity. While you want to challenge yourself, it's okay if you can't do all the recommended reps or sets at the start. Begin by trying to finish a single set of each exercise in the workout, then gradually work up to more as you progress. Within any set, only do as many reps as you can manage while following instructions, maintaining good form, and sticking to the specified tempo. If necessary, try lightening up the weight or resistance to make this possible.

3. How much weight or resistance should I use?

It's wise to have a selection of light weights (1, 2, and 3 pounds) and resistance tubing or bands (light through medium resistance).

Select the highest weight or level of resistance that allows you to accomplish all of the following:
- maintain good form throughout the exercise
- stick to the specified tempo
- complete the suggested number of reps and sets
- achieve a full and pain-free range of motion.

Wait until you find it easy to meet all four requirements before you increase the weight or resistance for a particular exercise. If it's difficult to meet any of the four, decrease the weight or resistance.

As you try the exercises, you'll find some muscle groups are stronger than other groups. Thus, you'll need to vary the amount of weight or resistance used in the course of your workout.

4. How often should I do the exercises in a workout?

A full workout incorporates warm-ups, muscle strengthening exercises, and stretches. We recommend doing full workouts two to three times a week. Strenuous exercise like strength training causes tiny tears in muscle tissue. The muscles grow stronger as the tears knit up. Always allow at least 48 hours between strength training sessions to give the muscles time to recover. Warm-ups and stretches can be done more often—even daily—to enhance flexibility.

5. How will I know I'm improving?

You can measure improvement in many ways. Before you launch your workouts, start by taking a few vital signs:

A. During a week, how often do you accumulate at least 30 minutes of moderate physical activity a day? Circle the number of days you achieve this:

0   1   2   3   4   5   6   7

Key: Ultimately, a healthy goal is achieving 150 minutes or more of moderate physical activity a week. It's perfectly fine to work up to that gradually. And remember, any activity is always better than none.

- **0–2 days:** See "A walking plan" on page 9 and focus on slow, steady gains.
- **3–4 days:** Great effort! If your time isn't adding up to 150 minutes or more weekly, try to shoehorn in brisk walks and similar activities on another day or two (see "When walks are too hard" on page 10 if you're looking for activities to try). Ten-minute chunks of activity are fine.
- **5+ days:** You've reached (or exceeded) your goal! Keep it up.

B. List three to five activities that are becoming more difficult to manage because of a low level of fitness or interference from a joint problem listed in our workouts—for example, a daily activity like walking up stairs, a task like reaching overhead to take a package off a high shelf, or a sports-related activity you enjoy.

1._____
2._____
3._____
4._____
5._____

Six weeks after starting your workouts, take a moment to reassess the physical activity vital signs that you wrote down. Notice any small leaps forward? Are you totting up more weekly minutes of activity or becoming active more days a week? Are the activities you listed becoming easier? If you're not quite there yet, applaud the strides you've made so far and keep trying.

6. When will I be ready to move on from a joint workout?

As long as you benefit from your workout, you may decide to stick with it. If you're itching to progress, though, you have several choices. When you can meet the four requirements described in question 3, do the following:

- Try the exercise variations under the "Too easy?" headings.
- Add weight or bump up resistance.
- Shift to a mainstream exercise program, preferably under the guidance of a personal trainer who can help you do this safely. ♥

Before you start the workouts: An important warning

Did you recently injure your ankle, knee, hip, wrist, elbow, or shoulder? Are you experiencing significant pain or discomfort in any of these joints? Have you had surgery on a joint? If so, it's vital to talk to your doctor before embarking on the workout directed at that particular joint.

Depending on the situation, you may receive the go-ahead or may need to rest and take other measures to heal properly first. In some instances, a doctor might want to modify certain exercises or may recommend working with a physical therapist.

If you think pain relief could help you exercise more comfortably, discuss the options with your doctor. Examples include the following:

Over-the-counter pain relievers. Naproxen (Aleve), ibuprofen (Advil), or acetaminophen (Tylenol) help reduce pain. Check with your doctor about the safest choice for you. Take 30 to 45 minutes before you do a workout.

Warm showers. Showering before exercise helps warm up muscles and joints.

Cold. Apply an ice wrap to the sore joint for 20 minutes after exercise.

Braces. When needed, a brace can help support muscles, distribute force, and limit movement. Talk to your doctor about whether a brace would be helpful, and, if so, which kind to choose.

Ankle workout

Your ankles must bear the full weight of your body, yet stay nimble and flexible. Every step, every jump, every dance move puts the ankle through a surprising range of motion. Even when you stand quietly, hips and knees at rest, the ankles are constantly moving and making minute adjustments to help you stay balanced.

Below you'll find brief descriptions of ankle anatomy (see Figure 1) and the joint problems that the ankle workout helps ease. The workout itself combines warm-ups, strength exercises to rebuild muscles that help protect your ankles, and stretches to release tight tendons, ligaments, and muscles.

Ankles 101

The large bone in the lower leg is the shin bone (tibia). It connects to the central ankle bone (talus). Bracketed by two bony bumps (each called a malleolus) on either side of the ankle, the talus acts as a hinge that allows you to point and flex your foot. Two other joints on the talus permit sideways movements. The shin bone bears all the weight; a second, smaller bone in the lower leg (fibula) ends alongside the talus. The heel bone (calcaneus) lies below the talus, cupping it. Two ligaments link the inner malleolus to the ankle bones. Three more ligaments bind the outer malleolus to the talus and calcaneus. Two large calf muscles, the gastrocnemius and soleus, are attached to the back of the foot by the strong, thick cord of the Achilles tendon. A muscle at the front of the shin (tibialis anterior) lifts the front of the foot, and the gastrocnemius lifts the heel.

What this workout helps

Chronic ankle sprains. Ankle sprains, an injury so common the American Academy of Orthopaedic Surgeons estimates it happens 25,000 times a day, occur when you roll your foot inward or outward, or turn or twist an ankle. That stretches, or even tears, the binding ligaments that keep the bones and joints properly positioned. Depending on the force applied as you land, the sprain can be mild, moderate, or severe. Chronic laxity in the ligaments makes repeated sprains more likely. While sports involving running, jumping, or sudden stops and turns sometimes play a role in sprains, they may also occur simply from crossing uneven ground or losing your balance.

Weak ankles. Weak muscles supporting the ankle affect balance and increase your vulnerability to injuries like sprains and falls.

Poor balance. Nerves in muscles and joints work with the vestibular system in your inner ear to constantly relay information about body movements and positioning. Called proprioception, this sixth sense operates independently of sight. By telling you where your ankle is in space, for example—stepping on a stair tread, perhaps, or recovering from a step onto uneven pavement—it helps you keep your balance. Like muscle strength, proprioception responds to training.

Figure 1 Ankle anatomy

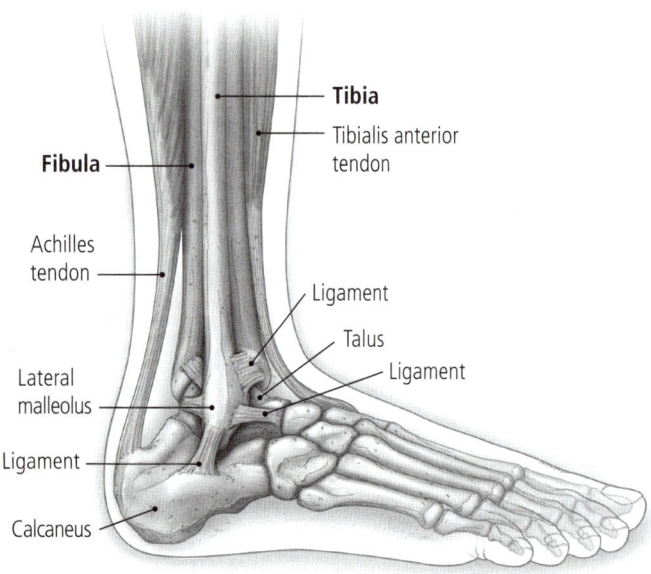

While standing, your ankle bears the full weight of your body and helps you stay balanced. The central ankle bone is the talus. The joint at this bone allows you to point and flex your foot while two other joints on the talus permit sideways movement.

Ankle exercises

Weak ankles often can be traced to repeated sprains that make the ligaments lax. This can set the stage for additional sprains or a fall that results in other injuries—possibly even broken bones.

This workout helps increase much-needed flexibility in your ankles and builds up supporting muscles that keep you balanced whether you're standing still, walking over changing terrain, or enjoying activities like dancing where you're moving in many directions. Plus, it enhances proprioception—the sense that tells you where your ankle is in space and helps you keep your balance. Ultimately, all of this can help prevent or limit falls.

We recommend performing the full workout two to three times a week. Make sure you leave 48 hours between strength exercise sessions to allow muscles time to recover. Warm-ups and stretches can be done daily to further enhance flexibility.

Equipment: Mat, resistance bands, sturdy chair, 1- to 3-pound ankle weights (optional), 3- to 5-pound dumbbells (optional).

Note: For this workout, take a length of resistance band and create a loop at one end of it, knotting it securely. Before each use, make sure there are no nicks or cuts in the band that could cause it to break.

1 WARMING UP: Ankle pumps

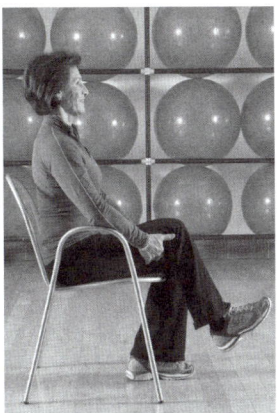 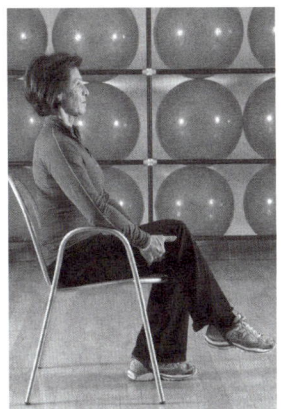

Reps: 10 **Sets:** 1
Intensity: Light
Tempo: Slow and controlled
Rest: No rest needed

Starting position: Sit up straight in a chair with your feet flat on the floor. Lift your right foot a few inches off the floor.

Movement: Flex your foot to point your toes toward the ceiling. Then point your foot and toes toward the floor. Finish all reps, then repeat with your left leg. This completes one set.

Tips and techniques:
- Maintain neutral posture with your shoulders down and back.
- Breathe comfortably.

Too hard? Make your movements smaller.

Too easy? Do two to three sets.

2 WARMING UP: Foot rotations

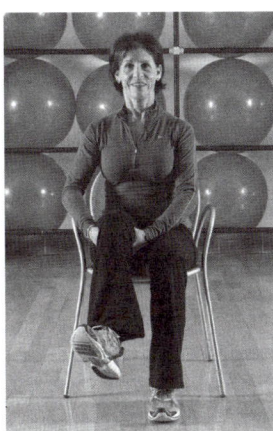 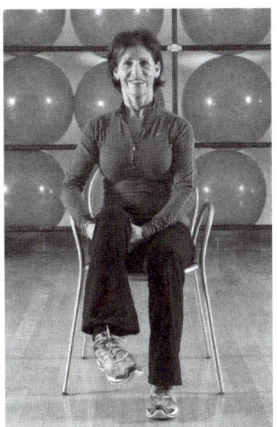

Reps: 10 in each direction **Sets:** 1
Intensity: Light
Tempo: Slow and controlled
Rest: No rest needed

Starting position: Sit up straight in a chair.

Movement: Lift your right foot off the floor. Rotate your foot from the ankle in a circle going clockwise. Finish all reps, then repeat foot rotations going counterclockwise. Repeat circles in both directions with your left foot. This completes one set.

Tips and techniques:
- Maintain neutral posture with your shoulders down and back.
- Breathe comfortably.

Too hard? Support your leg with both hands for assistance.

Too easy? Do two to three sets.

ANKLE WORKOUT

3 WARMING UP: Writing the alphabet

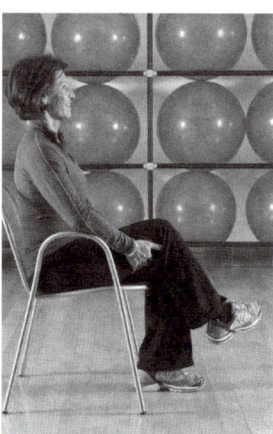 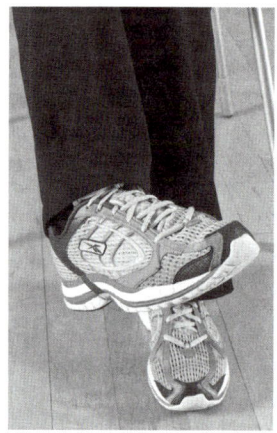

Reps: 1 per letter
Sets: 1
Intensity: Light
Tempo: Slow and controlled
Rest: No rest needed

Starting position: Sit up straight in a chair with your feet flat on the floor.

Movement: Lift your right foot a few inches off the floor and use your toes to write the alphabet in the air. The writing motions should come from the ankle. Repeat with the toes on your left foot. This completes one set.

Tips and techniques:
- Maintain neutral posture with your shoulders down and back.
- Breathe comfortably.

Too hard? Support your leg with both hands for assistance.
Too easy? Do two to three sets.

4 STRENGTHENING: Single leg stance

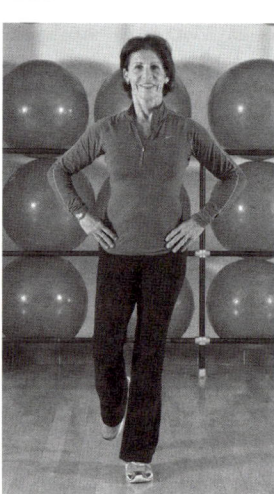

Reps: 1 per leg   **Sets:** 1–3
Intensity: Moderate to hard
Hold: 60 seconds
Rest: 30–90 seconds between sets

Starting position: Stand up straight with your feet hip-width apart.

Movement: Lift your right foot a few inches off the floor, bending your knee slightly, and balancing on your left leg. Hold for 60 seconds, then lower your foot to the starting position. Repeat with your left leg. This completes one set.

Tips and techniques:
- Maintain neutral posture with your shoulders down and back.
- Tighten the muscles around your hips and buttocks for stability.
- Keep your abdominal muscles contracted.

Too hard? Hold on to a chair or counter for support, or perform for less than 60 seconds.
Too easy? Stand on a soft mat to make it more difficult to balance.

5 STRENGTHENING: Heel raises

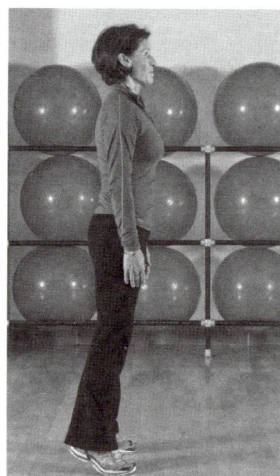

Reps: 10
Sets: 1–3
Intensity: Light to moderate
Tempo: 3-1-3
Rest: 30–90 seconds between sets

Starting position: Stand up straight with your feet hip-width apart and your hands at your sides.

Movement: Slowly lift up on your toes so that your heels rise off the floor as high as possible. Pause, then slowly return to the starting position.

Tips and techniques:
- Maintain neutral posture with your shoulders down and back.
- Stand evenly on your toes and heels before lifting and when returning to the starting position.
- Exhale as you lift.

Too hard? Hold on to a chair or counter for support.
Too easy? Hold weights (3 to 5 pounds) in your hands while doing the exercise.

ANKLE WORKOUT

6 STRENGTHENING: Point and flex

Reps: 10 **Sets:** 1–3
Intensity: Moderate
Tempo: 3-1-3
Rest: 30–90 seconds between sets

Starting position: Sit up straight in a chair with your feet flat on the floor. Extend your right leg with toes pointing toward the ceiling. Put the resistance band loop around the ball of your right foot like a sling. Hold the other end with both hands, keeping tension on it throughout the exercise.

Movement: This is a two-step exercise.
Step 1: Slowly point your foot toward the floor, pause, then slowly return to the starting position. Finish all reps.
Step 2: Place your right ankle on top of your left knee. Put the loop just below your right toes on top of the foot, keeping tension on this with your left hand. Slowly pull the toes of your right foot upward toward your right shin, pause, then slowly return to the Step 2 starting position. Finish all reps. Now repeat both steps with your left foot. This completes one set.

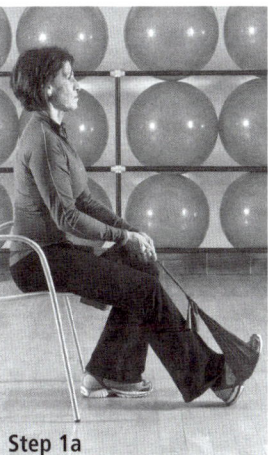
Step 1a

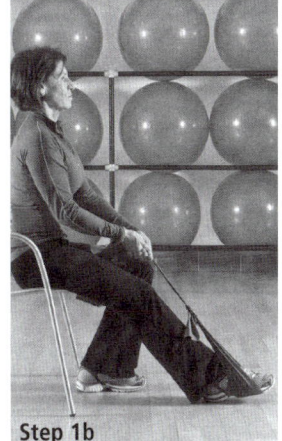
Step 1b

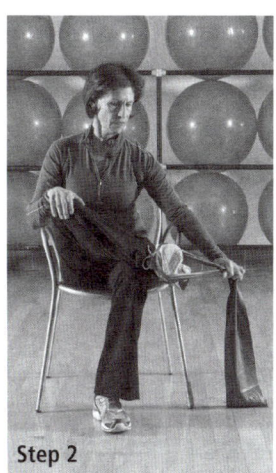
Step 2

Tips and techniques:
- Keep tension on the band at all times to create resistance.
- Maintain neutral posture with your shoulders down and back.
- Breathe comfortably.

Too hard? Use a lighter resistance band.
Too easy? Use a heavier resistance band.

7 STRENGTHENING: Inversion and eversion

Reps: 10 **Sets:** 1–3
Intensity: Moderate
Tempo: 3-1-3
Rest: 30–90 seconds between sets

Starting position: Sit on a mat with your legs extended. Bend your right knee and put the foot flat on the floor. Lift the toes toward the ceiling and place the loop of the resistance band around the ball of your right foot. Hold the band in your right hand, keeping tension on it.

Movement: This is a two-step exercise with a side-to-side movement. *Step 1:* Slowly turn your right foot inward. Pause, then return to center. Finish all reps. *Step 2:* Hold the band in your left hand, keeping tension on it. Slowly turn your right foot outward. Pause, then return to center. Finish all reps. Then repeat both steps with the loop on your left foot. This completes one set.

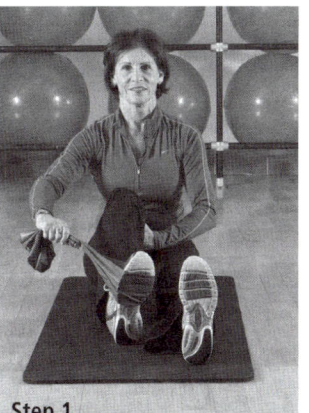
Step 1

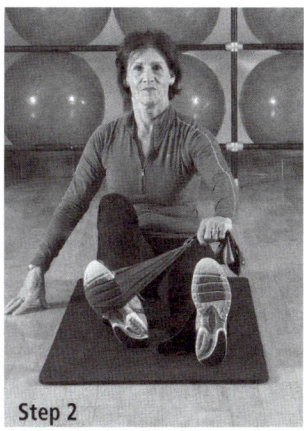
Step 2

Tips and techniques:
- Keep tension on the band at all times to create resistance.
- Keep your heel on the floor throughout both steps.
- Maintain neutral posture with your shoulders down and back.

Too hard? Sit against a wall and use a lighter resistance band.
Too easy? Use a heavier resistance band.

ANKLE WORKOUT

8 STRENGTHENING: Toe taps

Reps: 10 front, 10 side-to-side **Sets:** 1–3
Intensity: Light to moderate
Tempo: 1-1
Rest: 30–90 seconds between sets

Starting position: Stand up straight with your hands on your hips and your feet hip-width apart. Move your right foot forward so the right heel is in line with the toes of your left foot.

Movement: This is a two-step exercise. *Step 1:* While keeping your heel grounded on the floor, lift the toes of your right foot as high as you can and tap them on the floor 10 times.
Step 2: Still keeping your heel grounded, lift up the toes of your right foot, then tap in and out (to the left and right) 10 times. Repeat both steps with your left foot. This completes one set.

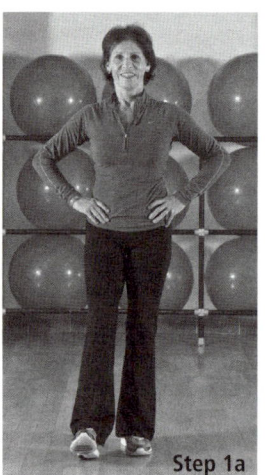
Step 1a

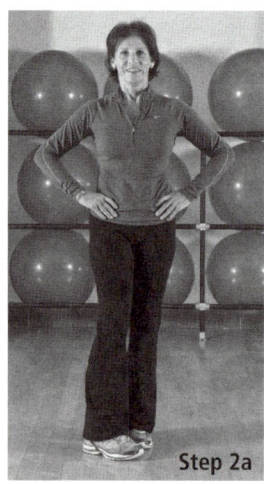
Step 2a

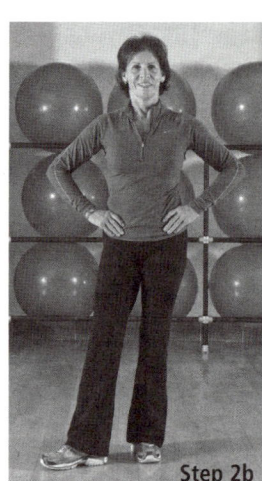
Step 2b

Tips and techniques:
- Maintain neutral posture with your shoulders down and back.
- Keep toe taps smooth and controlled.

Too hard? Perform the exercise while seated in a chair with both feet on the floor.

Too easy? Secure a 1- to 3-pound ankle weight around your foot behind the toes.

9 STRETCHING: Standing lower calf stretch

Reps: 3–4
Sets: 1
Intensity: Light
Hold: 10–30 seconds
Rest: No rest needed

Starting position: Stand up straight in front of a wall with your arms extended at shoulder height.

Movement: Place your hands on the wall. Extend your right leg straight back and press the heel toward the floor. Let your left leg bend as you do so. Hold. Return to the starting position, then repeat with your left leg. This is one rep. Continue alternating feet until you finish all reps.

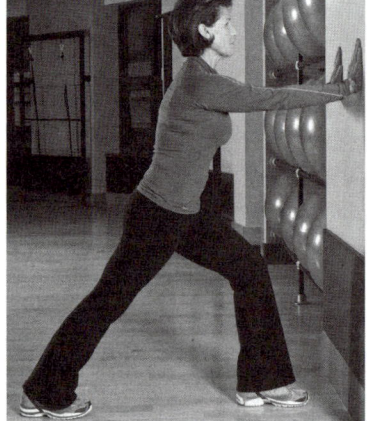

Tips and techniques:
- Stretch to the point of mild tension, not pain.
- Hold a full-body lean from the ankle as you stretch.
- Maintain neutral posture with your shoulders down and back.

Too hard? Hold the back of a chair and do not press as far into the stretch.

Too easy? Try to bend your back knee farther without lifting your heel off the floor. This increases the stretch.

10 STRETCHING: Standing soleus stretch

Reps: 3–4 **Sets:** 1
Intensity: Light
Hold: 10–30 seconds
Rest: No rest needed

Starting position: Stand up straight in front of a wall with your arms extended at shoulder height.

Movement: Place your hands on the wall. Extend your right leg straight back and press the heel toward the floor. Let your left knee bend slightly as you do so, while keeping the heel grounded on the floor. Now bend your right knee as much as possible without lifting the heel off the floor. Hold. Return to the starting position. Finish all reps, then repeat with your left foot. This completes the set.

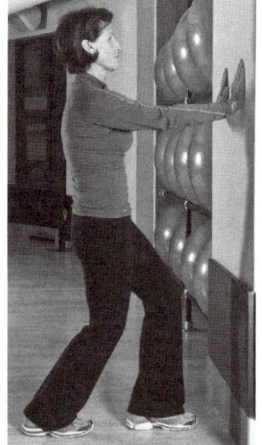

Tips and techniques:
- Stretch to the point of mild tension, not pain.
- Hold a full-body lean from the ankle as you stretch.
- Maintain neutral posture with your shoulders down and back.

Too hard? Hold the back of a chair and do not press as far into the stretch.

Too easy? Try to bend your back knee farther without lifting your heel off the floor. This increases the stretch.

ANKLE WORKOUT

11 STRETCHING: Inversion and eversion ankle stretch

Reps: 3–4
Sets: 1
Intensity: Light
Hold: 10–30 seconds
Rest: No rest needed

Starting position: Sit in a chair with your feet flat on the floor.

Movement: This is a side-to-side movement. Lift your entire right foot a few inches off the floor. Slowly bring the toes of your right foot inward. Hold. Return to center, then slowly bring the toes of your right foot outward to complete one rep. Hold. Finish all reps, then repeat the stretch with your left foot.

Tips and techniques:
- Stretch to the point of mild tension, not pain.
- Maintain neutral posture with your shoulders down and back.
- Breathe comfortably.

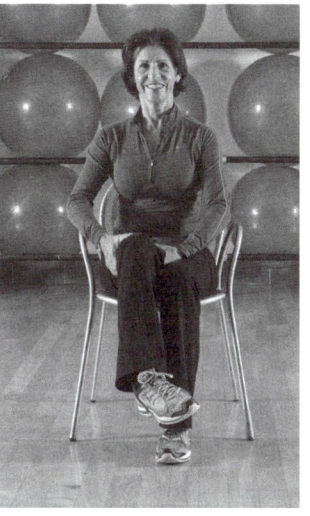
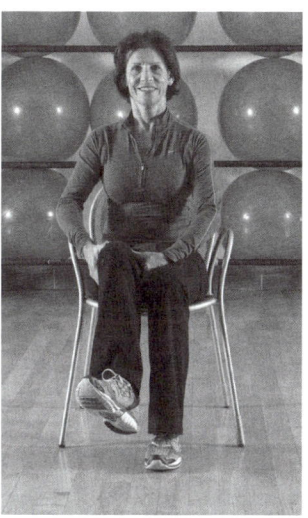

Too hard? Keep your heel grounded on the floor as you turn your foot inward or outward in the stretch.

Too easy? Repeat the stretch several times throughout the day.

12 STRETCHING: Seated point and flex

Reps: 3–4
Sets: 1
Intensity: Light
Hold: 10–30 seconds
Rest: No rest needed

Starting position: Sit up straight in a chair with both feet on the floor.

Movement: Lift your right foot a few inches off the floor. Slowly flex your ankle so your toes point up toward the ceiling. Hold. Then slowly point your toes toward the floor. Hold. Finish all reps, then repeat the stretch with your left foot. This completes the set.

Tips and techniques:
- Stretch to the point of mild tension, not pain.
- Maintain neutral posture with your shoulders down and back.
- Breathe comfortably.

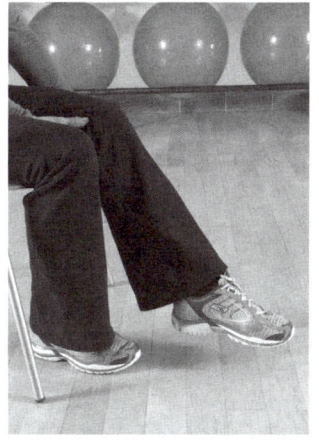
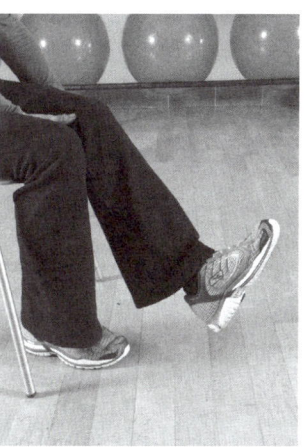

Too hard? Try the stretch while lying on your back with legs extended, so that the backs of your heels touch the floor. Slowly flex your toes and both feet back toward your shin as far as possible. Hold. Slowly point your toes and feet. Hold. This is one rep.

Too easy? Repeat the stretch several times throughout the day.

Note: Special thanks to the Equinox fitness club at 131 Dartmouth Street in Boston for the use of its facilities, and to the following Equinox personal trainers, instructors, and staff members for demonstrating the exercises depicted in this report: Kristy DiScipio, Josie Gardiner, Tracey Knox, and Hector Mancebo.

Knee workout

"Oil me," begged the Tin Man haltingly. "Oil me." None of us is made of enough metal to rust in the rain, but creaky, painful knees may make you wish there was such a simple solution. While there isn't, there are some things you can do to ease knee pain and build up surrounding muscles so they better support your knee.

Below you'll find brief descriptions of knee anatomy (see Figure 2) and joint problems that the knee workout helps ease. The workout itself combines warm-ups, strength exercises to rebuild muscles that help protect your knees, and stretches to release tight tendons, ligaments, and muscles.

Knees 101

The largest joint in the body is the knee. It acts as a hinge that allows your lower leg and foot to swing easily forward or back as you walk, run, or kick. A healthy knee allows almost 150 degrees of movement. But unlike a simple hinge like one on a jewelry box, for example, in which any wobble is undesirable, the knee can slightly rotate or move from side to side, as well. To form the joint, knuckles at the lower end of the thighbone (femur) fit smoothly into dimples in the upper end of the shin bone (tibia) formed by cushioning layers of cartilage called menisci. A quartet of ligaments knits the bones together: a pair of stretchy cruciate ligaments in the interior, and a pair of collateral ligaments on the outer sides of the joint. The kneecap (patella) covers the front of the joint. A large connecting tendon bridges the shin, the kneecap, and the large four-part muscle at the front of the thigh called the quadriceps.

What this workout helps

■ **Osteoarthritis.** This condition is sometimes dubbed "wear and tear" arthritis because it starts when cartilage cushioning the joints wears down (see Figure 3). Tenderness and morning pain or stiffness that lasts less than 30 minutes are telltale signs of this condition. Osteoarthritis of the knee affects more than four million Americans over age 60. Prior injuries, excess weight, aging, and overuse are among the factors that set the stage for knee osteoarthritis. Interestingly, findings from the Framingham Offspring Cohort study suggest that moderately intense exercise like walking or running—at least on normal knees—does not increase the likelihood of osteoarthritis.

■ **Bursitis.** Small fluid-filled sacs called bursae cushion the movement of bones against muscle, skin, and tendons. Inflammation of a bursa is known as bursitis. Two prime candidates for bursitis lie above and below the knee. Prolonged kneeling while gardening or performing tasks, or sustaining a direct hit to the front of the knee during sports or an accident, can cause bursitis. Tight hamstring muscles, certain anatomical fac-

Figure 2 Strong and flexible

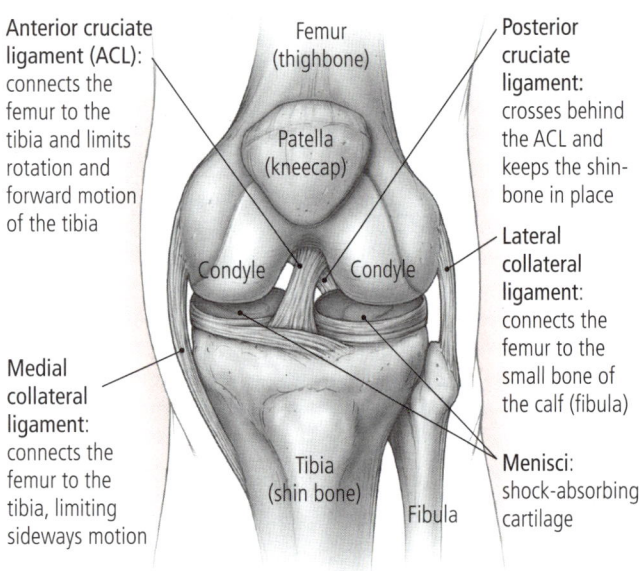

The knee is more than a simple hinge. Along with the strength to raise and lower your body weight, this joint also has supporting structures to allow you to twist and turn.

tors, or actions like repeatedly kicking a ball may play into it, too.

■ **Tendinitis.** Marked by pain and swelling above or below the kneecap where tendons attach to bone, tendinitis (inflamed tendons) may have many causes. As you age, protective muscles like the quadriceps weaken and tendons become less flexible. "Weekend warriors" may pay the price for engaging in high-intensity activities like basketball, tennis, or squash without being properly conditioned. Vigorous, repetitive use—or rather overuse—of tendons brought on by dancing, running, or jumping is another possibility.

■ **Runner's knee (patellofemoral pain syndrome).** When quadriceps and hamstrings—muscles at the front and back of the thighs—are not sufficiently strong, runners may bend less at the knee while exercising. This funnels pressure to a smaller area, prompting overuse damage that may cause osteoarthritis over time.

Figure 3 Osteoarthritis of the knee

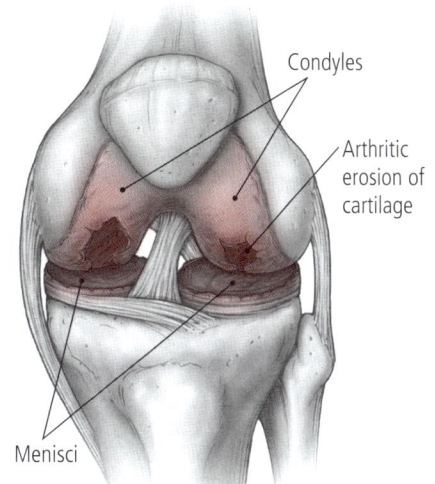

Age, mechanical wear and tear, genetics, and biochemical factors all contribute to the gradual degeneration of the cartilage and the menisci. In this illustration, the cartilage of the condyles (knobs at the lower end of the thighbone) is degraded.

Knee exercises

Strengthening muscles around the knee and maintaining their power reduces stress across the joint. This workout will help you improve flexibility around your knee and build up supporting muscles. If you have osteoarthritis of the knee—a very common complaint as years roll by—doing so will help keep you mobile. Further, building adequate strength and flexibility around the knee makes you less susceptible to bursitis and tendinitis.

We recommend performing the full workout two to three times a week. Make sure you leave 48 hours between strength exercise sessions to allow muscles time to recover. However, warm-ups and stretches can be done daily to further enhance flexibility.

Equipment: Mat, sturdy chair, stability ball, 1- to 3-pound ankle weights (optional), yoga strap (optional).

---

1 | WARMING UP: **Walk forward and back**

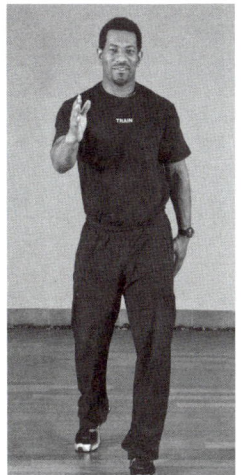

Reps: 10 steps in each direction
Sets: 1–3
Intensity: Light
Tempo: Slow and controlled
Rest: No rest needed

Starting position: Stand up straight with your arms by your sides.
Movement: Walk 10 steps forward. Walk 10 steps backward. This completes one set.

Tips and techniques:
- Maintain neutral posture with your shoulders down and back.
- Let your arms swing naturally forward and back.

KNEE WORKOUT

2 WARMING UP: Mini-squats

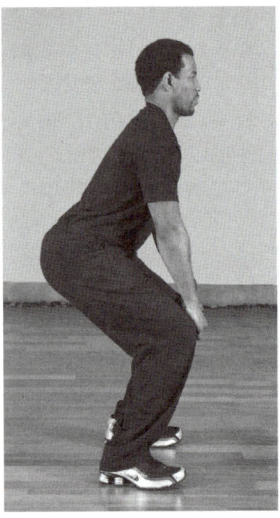

Reps: 10
Sets: 1–3
Intensity: Moderate
Tempo: Slow and controlled
Rest: No rest needed

Starting position: Stand up straight with your feet hip-width apart.

Movement: Rest your hands on your thighs. Hinge forward at your hips and bend your knees to lower your buttocks about six inches, as if starting to sit down in a chair. Return to the starting position.

Tips and techniques:
- Press your weight back into your heels when squatting.
- Keep your knees aligned over your ankles and pointing forward as you squat.
- Keep your spine neutral and your shoulders down and back.

Too hard? Do a smaller squat.
Too easy? Hold each mini-squat for eight counts.

3 WARMING UP: Alternating hamstring curls

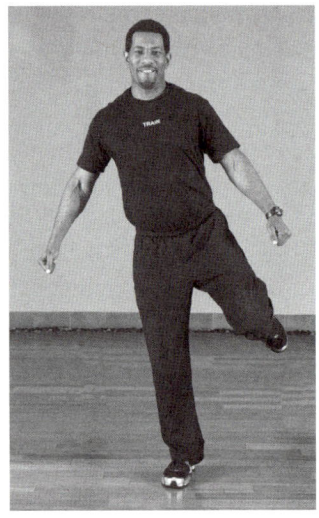

Reps: 10
Sets: 1–3
Intensity: Light
Tempo: Slow and controlled
Rest: No rest needed

Starting position: Stand up straight with your feet hip-width apart.

Movement: Lift your right heel toward your buttocks and return to the starting position, then lift your left heel toward your buttocks and return to the starting position. This is one rep.

Tips and techniques:
- Maintain neutral posture with your shoulders down and back.
- Contract your abdominal muscles.
- Breathe naturally.

Too hard? Do not lift your heels as high.
Too easy? Add a little squat between lifts.

4 WARMING UP: Standing single leg circles

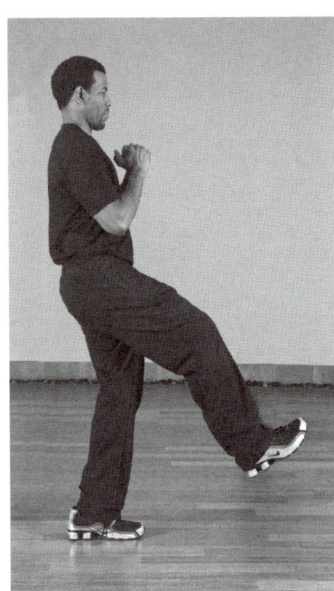

Reps: 10 per leg
Sets: 1–3
Intensity: Light
Tempo: Slow and controlled
Rest: No rest needed

Starting position: Stand up straight with your feet hip-width apart.
Movement: Lift your right foot off the floor and perform 10 leg circles as if pedaling a bike. Return to the starting position, then repeat with the left foot. This completes one set.

Tips and techniques:
- Maintain neutral posture with your shoulders down and back.
- Be sure to contract the buttock muscles in the standing hip for stability.
- Contract your abdominal muscles.

Too hard? Hold on to a chair or counter for support.
Too easy? Try not to touch the floor as you make each circular motion.

KNEE WORKOUT

5 STRENGTHENING: Supine knee extension

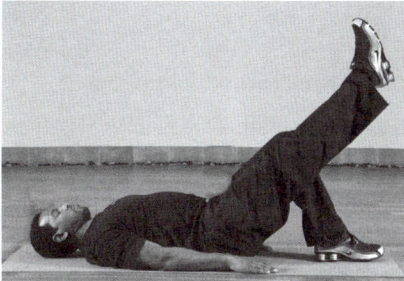

Reps: 10
Sets: 1–3
Intensity: Light to moderate
Tempo: 3-1-3
Rest: 30–90 seconds between sets

Starting position: Lie on a mat on your back with both knees bent and feet flat on the floor. Rest your arms at your sides.

Movement: Slowly lift your right foot off the floor and straighten your leg while keeping your knees level. Pause, then slowly lower your foot to the starting position so that both feet are flat on the floor. Finish all reps, then repeat with the left foot. This completes one set.

Tips and techniques:
- As you lift your foot, straighten your leg as much as possible without locking the knee.
- Maintain neutral posture with your shoulders down and back.
- Exhale as you lift.

Too hard? Lift your foot a shorter distance.
Too easy? Add a 1- to 3-pound ankle weight.

6 STRENGTHENING: Seated knee extension

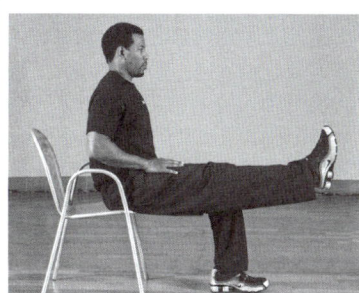

Reps: 10 per leg
Sets: 1–3
Intensity: Light to moderate
Tempo: 3-1-3
Rest: 30–90 seconds between sets

Starting position: Sit up straight on a chair or bench with your feet flat on the floor and your hands resting on your thighs.

Movement: Slowly lift up your right foot to the level of your hip. Pause, then slowly lower the foot to the starting position (flat on the floor). Finish all reps, then repeat with the left leg. This completes one set.

Tips and techniques:
- Maintain neutral posture with your shoulders down and back.
- Lift your leg as high as possible without locking your knee.
- Exhale as you lift.

Too hard? Lift your foot a shorter distance.
Too easy? Add a 1- to 3-pound ankle weight.

7 STRENGTHENING: Chair stand with staggered legs

Reps: 10 per leg   **Sets:** 1–3
Intensity: Moderate to hard
Tempo: 3-1-3
Rest: 30–90 seconds between sets

Starting position: Sit up straight near the front edge of a chair with your arms crossed and fingers touching opposite shoulders. Position your feet hip-width apart and stagger them by moving your right foot forward.

Movement: Smoothly stand up with your knees and hips pointing straight ahead. Pause, then return to the starting position. Finish all reps before repeating with the left foot forward. This completes one set.

Tips and techniques:
- Maintain neutral posture throughout the movement.
- Tighten the muscles in your abdomen and buttocks.
- Exhale as you lift up.

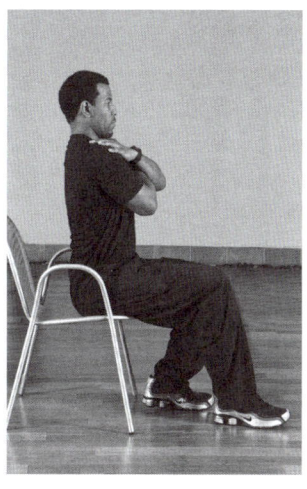 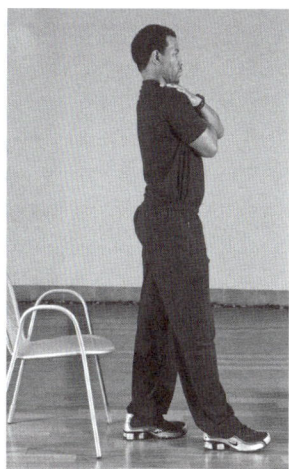

Too hard? Line up your feet evenly, hip-width apart, in the starting position.

Too easy? Lift your arms over your head. Keep your shoulders down and back throughout the move.

KNEE WORKOUT

8 STRENGTHENING: Single leg lift

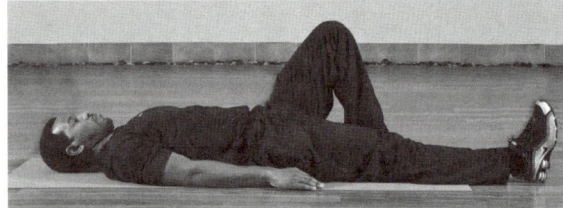

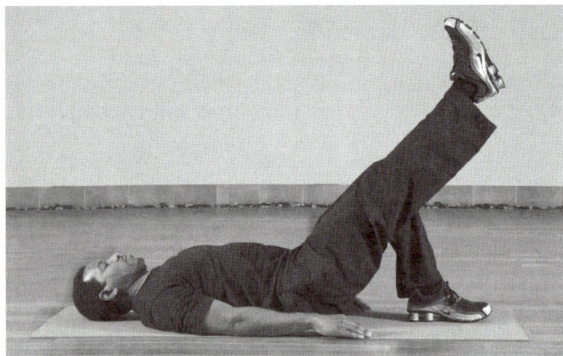

Reps: 10 per leg **Sets:** 1–3
Intensity: Light to moderate
Tempo: 3-1-3   **Rest:** 30–90 seconds between sets

Starting position: Lie on your back with your left knee bent and foot flat on the floor. Extend your right leg. Rest your hands by your hips on the floor.

Movement: Tighten your thigh muscles and slowly lift your right leg in the air to the height of your left knee. Pause, then slowly lower your leg to rest on the floor. Finish all reps, then repeat with the left leg. This completes one set.

Tips and techniques:
- Maintain neutral posture with your shoulders down and back.
- Be sure to tighten your thigh muscle before lifting the leg.
- Exhale as you lift.

Too hard? Lift your leg a shorter distance.

Too easy? Try doing the leg lift in the shape of a T at a slow, controlled pace. Lift up your right leg 4 inches, move the leg toward your left leg 4 inches, return to center, move the leg 4 inches to the right, return to center, then lower your leg to the floor. Finish all reps, then repeat with the left leg. This completes one set.

9 STRENGTHENING: Wall squats with stability ball

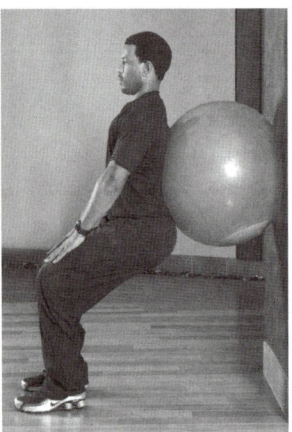

Reps: 10 **Sets:** 1–3
Intensity: Moderate to hard
Tempo: 3-1-3
Rest: 30–90 seconds between sets

Starting position: Stand up straight and place the stability ball between the back of your waist and the wall. Walk your feet out about 18 to 24 inches, while keeping the ball at waist height. Rest your hands on your thighs.

Movement: Slowly bend your knees and hips into a squat as if you were sitting down in a chair. (The ball will roll up your back as you move downward.) Stop before your buttocks reach knee level. Slowly straighten your legs as you return to the starting position.

Tips and techniques:
- Maintain neutral posture with your shoulders down and back.
- Keep your knees aligned over your ankles and pointing forward as you squat.
- Exhale as you return to the starting position.

Too hard? Do a smaller squat.
Too easy? Hold each squat for eight counts.

10 STRETCHING: Quadriceps stretch on stomach

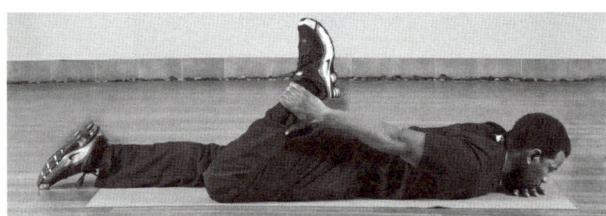

Reps: 3–4 per leg **Sets:** 1 **Intensity:** Moderate
Hold: 10–30 seconds **Rest:** No rest needed

Starting position: Lie on your stomach on the floor with your hands flat under your chin.

Movement: Bend your right knee and try to bring the heel toward your right buttock. Reach back with your right hand and take hold of your foot. Hold the stretch, then slowly lower your foot to the floor. Repeat the stretch with your left leg. Continue alternating legs until you finish all reps.

Tips and techniques:
- Stretch to the point of mild tension, not pain.
- Breathe comfortably.

Too hard? Place a yoga strap around your foot to assist with the stretch.

Too easy? Lift your knee up slightly off the floor to increase the stretch.

11 STRETCHING: Alternating hamstring stretch

Reps: 3–4 **Sets:** 1
Intensity: Moderate to hard
Hold: 10–30 seconds **Rest:** No rest needed

Starting position: Lie on your back with both knees bent and feet flat on the floor.

Movement: Grasp your right leg with both hands behind the thigh. Extend your leg to lift your right foot toward the ceiling. Straighten the leg as much as possible without locking the knee and flex the ankle to stretch the calf muscles. Hold. Return to the starting position and repeat with the left leg. This completes one rep.

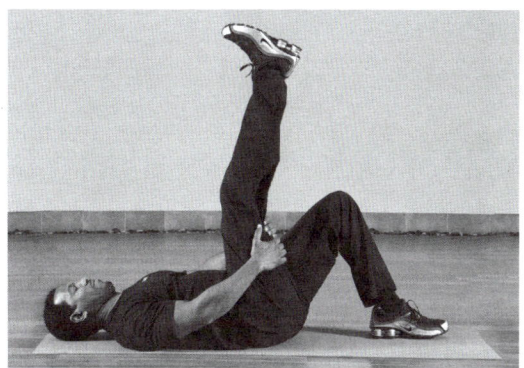

Tips and techniques:

- Stretch the leg extended toward the ceiling to the point of mild tension without any pressure behind the knee or any pain.
- Relax your shoulders down and back into the floor.
- Breathe comfortably.

Too hard? Sit up straight in a chair and extend your right leg straight out in front of you with the heel grounded on the floor and the toes pointing to the ceiling. Hinge forward from the hip while maintaining a neutral spine. Hold. Repeat with the left leg. This completes one rep.

Too easy? Stand upright and extend your right leg straight in front of you with your foot on a chair or counter. Flex your ankle. Hinge forward from the hip while maintaining a neutral spine. Hold. Repeat with the left leg. This completes one rep.

Hip workout

Ever seen children spin hula hoops in easy, endless gyrations? Or watched the tiny, shivering moves made by a belly dancer with one hip aslant? Remember doing the Twist? Then you know that hips are capable of far more than most of us manage in the course of our daily rounds. If you have hip pain, you may not be doing the Twist soon, but by conditioning the muscles that help support your hip, you may find that you can perform physical activities and everyday tasks more easily and painlessly.

This section includes brief descriptions of hip anatomy (see Figure 4) and joint and muscle problems that the hip workout helps ease. The workout moves from warm-ups to strength exercises aimed at rebuilding muscles that help protect your hips. Stretches help release tight tendons and muscles that affect gait and balance and may play a role in back pain, too.

Figure 4 Hip anatomy

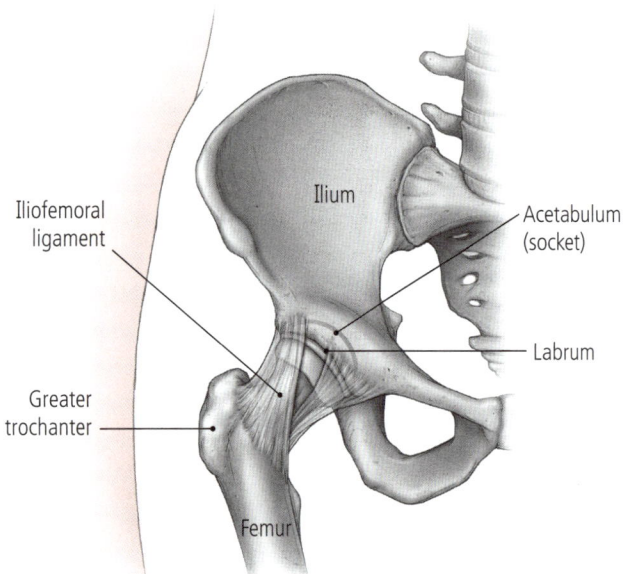

The hip is a ball-and-socket joint reinforced by a strong ring of cartilage (labrum) inside the socket (acetabulum). Supporting ligaments allow for a wide range of motion while the hip bears the full weight of the upper body.

Hips 101

The hip joint is a ball-and-socket design, albeit one with far less flexibility than the shoulder joint. Three fused bones—the ischium, ilium, and pubis—shape the basin of the pelvis. At the neck of the thighbone (femur), a bump branches off to form the ball of the hip joint with its cushioning layer of cartilage. The ball fits snugly into a socket in the pelvis (acetabulum). Thanks to the perfect fit, along with the slick cartilage coating the bones and the fluid lubricating the space between them, the friction between the ball and socket in a healthy hip is less than that of two ice cubes rubbing together. A larger projection slightly lower on the thighbone provides an anchor for tendons that run into leg and hip muscles, while a series of ligaments tightly binds the joint to help provide stability.

What this workout helps

■ **Osteoarthritis.** Sometimes dubbed "wear and tear" arthritis because it starts when cartilage cushioning the joints wears down, osteoarthritis of the hip affects approximately 10 million American adults. The joint space narrows and the cartilage thins as bones rub against it, or eventually against each other, sometimes to the point of creating rough spots or bone spurs. Marked by pain in the groin or down the leg, this condition may go unreported because people sometimes assume that the knee, rather than the hip, is the problem. Prior injuries, excess weight, aging, and overuse are among the factors that set the stage for hip osteoarthritis.

■ **Poor balance.** Muscles known as hip flexors allow you to bend at the hip and bring your knee up toward your chest. Often, these muscles grow tight and shorten, tugging your upper body forward. This affects balance and gait while walking.

■ **Back pain.** Short, tight hip flexors contribute to lower back pain, particularly when the iliopsoas muscles, which balance your pelvis, are tight, too.

HIP WORKOUT

Hip exercises

By enhancing hip flexibility and strengthening supporting muscles, this workout improves balance and makes walking easier. It also helps address pain and reduced mobility from osteoarthritis of the hip, as well as back pain.

We recommend performing the full workout two to three times a week. Make sure you leave 48 hours between strength exercise sessions to allow muscles time to recover. However, warm-ups and stretches can be done daily, if you wish, to further enhance flexibility.

Equipment: Mat, stability ball, yoga strap, sturdy chair (optional), resistance tubing (optional), 1- to 3-pound ankle weights (optional).

---

1 WARMING UP: Alternating knee lifts

Reps: 10
Sets: 1
Intensity: Light
Tempo: Slow and controlled
Rest: No rest needed

Starting position: Stand up straight with your feet together and your hands at your sides.

Movement: Lift your right knee toward the ceiling. Lower to the starting position. Repeat with your left knee. This is one rep.

Tips and techniques:
- Keep your chest lifted and your shoulders down and back.
- Contract your abdominal muscles throughout.

Too hard? Hold on to a chair for support.

Too easy? Do 10 knee lifts on the right side, then 10 on the left, to complete one set.

---

2 WARMING UP: Hip circles on stability ball

Reps: 10 in both directions   **Sets:** 1
Intensity: Light   **Tempo:** Slow and controlled
Rest: No rest needed

Starting position: Sit on a stability ball with your feet hip-width apart. Place your hands next to your hips on the ball for extra support.

Movement: Make 10 slow, circular movements with your hips clockwise to loosen up your hip joints, keeping your buttocks on the ball as you do so. Repeat counterclockwise.

Tips and techniques:
- Maintain neutral posture with your shoulders down and back.
- Contract your abdominal muscles throughout.
- Keep your pace slow and controlled.

---

3 WARMING UP: Hip circles on back

Reps: 20 per leg
Sets: 1
Intensity: Light
Tempo: Slow and controlled
Rest: No rest needed

Starting position: Lie on your back with your left knee bent and the foot flat on the floor. Place a yoga strap over the foot of the right leg and extend it.

Movement: Point the toes of your right foot slightly toward the ceiling and slowly make 10 small circles to the right. Then make 10 small circles to the left. Repeat with the left leg.

Tips and techniques:
- Initiate the movement from the hip.
- Contract your abdominal muscles and be sure your back is touching the floor throughout.

Too hard? Make smaller circles to limit your range of motion.
Too easy? Make larger circles.

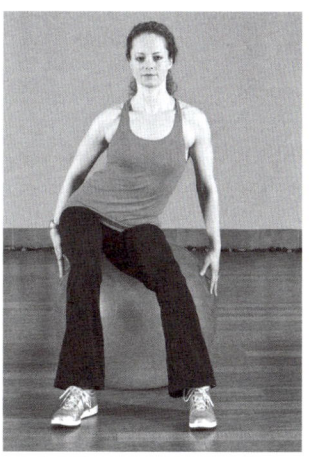
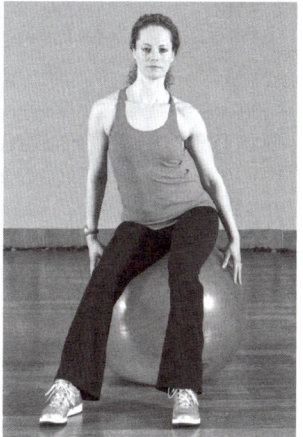

Too hard? Perform hip circles standing upright with knees slightly bent.

Too easy? Perform the exercise without holding on to the ball.

---

www.health.harvard.edu   The Joint Pain Relief Workout   31

HIP WORKOUT

4 STRENGTHENING: Side-lying clam

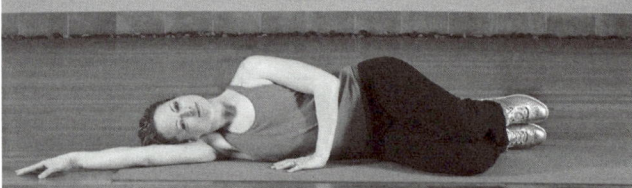
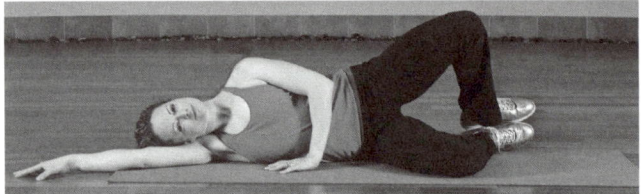

Reps: 10 per leg **Sets:** 1–3
Intensity: Light to moderate **Tempo:** 3-1-3
Rest: 30–90 seconds between sets

Starting position: Lie on your right side, knees bent so your heels are in line with your buttocks. Rest your head on your right arm on the floor.

Movement: Keep your feet together as you slowly lift your left knee up toward the ceiling. Pause, then slowly return to the starting position. Finish all reps, then repeat on the left side. This completes one set.

Tips and techniques:
- Throughout the movement, keep your hips stacked and still as if you were lying with your back against a wall.
- Lift your top knee up as high as possible without letting your hip move.
- Exhale as you lift.

Too hard? Lift your top knee a shorter distance.
Too easy? Tie resistance tubing around your upper thighs above your knees, or increase the number of reps.

5 STRENGTHENING: Wall squats with stability ball

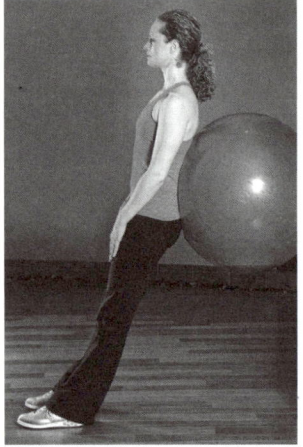
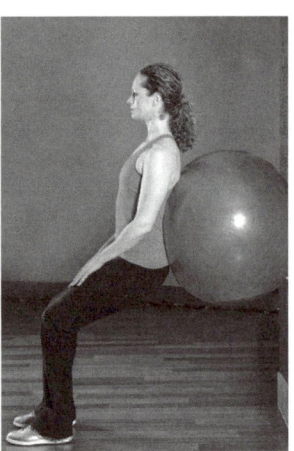

Reps: 10 **Sets:** 1–3
Intensity: Moderate **Tempo:** 3-1-3
Rest: 30–90 seconds between sets

Starting position: Stand up straight and place the stability ball between the back of your waist and the wall. Walk your feet out about 18 to 24 inches, while keeping the ball at waist height. Rest your hands on your thighs.

Movement: Slowly bend your knees and hips into a squat as if you were sitting down in a chair. (The ball will roll up your back as you move downward.) Stop before your buttocks reach knee level. Straighten your legs as you return to the starting position.

Tips and techniques:
- Maintain neutral posture with your shoulders down and back.
- Keep your knees aligned over your ankles and pointing forward as you squat.
- Exhale as you return to the starting position.

Too hard? Do a smaller squat.
Too easy? Hold each squat for eight counts.

6 STRENGTHENING: Standing side leg lift

Reps: 10 per leg **Sets:** 1–3
Intensity: Moderate
Tempo: 3-1-3
Rest: 30–90 seconds between sets

Starting position: Stand up straight with your feet together and your hands on your hips.

Movement: Slowly lift your left leg straight out to the side. Pause, then slowly lower the leg. Keep your hips even throughout. Finish all reps, then repeat with the right leg. This completes one set.

Tips and techniques:
- Maintain neutral posture with your shoulders down and back.
- Tighten your abdominal muscles and squeeze the buttocks of your supporting leg.
- Exhale as you lift.

Too hard? Hold on to the back of a chair for balance and lift your leg a shorter distance.
Too easy? Hold for four counts at the top of the lift during each rep.

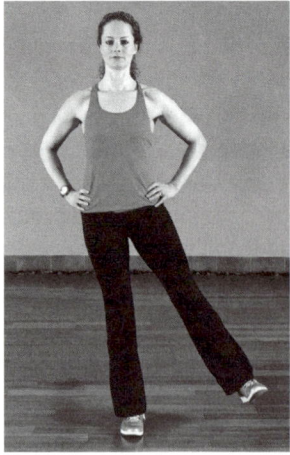

HIP WORKOUT

7 STRENGTHENING: Bridge with alternating single leg lift

Reps: 5 per leg
Sets: 1–3
Intensity: Moderate
Tempo: 2-2-2-2
Rest: 30–90 seconds between sets

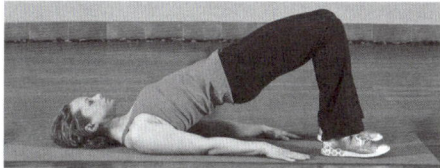
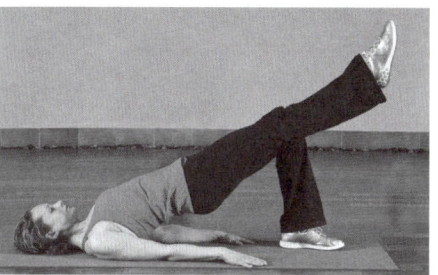

Starting position: Lie on your back on the floor with your knees bent and feet flat on the floor, hip-width apart. Place your arms at your sides. Relax your shoulders down and back against the floor.

Movement: Squeeze your buttocks as you lift your hips off the floor to a count of two. This is the bridge position. Lift the right foot and extend your leg out to the height of the bent knee to a count of two. Bring the right foot back to the floor into the bridge position to a count of two, then return to the starting position (hips on the floor) to a count of two. Repeat with the left leg. Continue alternating legs until you finish all reps. This completes one set.

Tips and techniques:
- Be sure to squeeze your buttocks before you lift up into the bridge position.
- Keep your shoulders, hips, and knees aligned.
- Relax your shoulders down and back into the floor.

Too hard? Perform the bridge without the leg extension, using a 2-1-2 count (lifting your hips up to a count of two, holding for one second, and returning your hips to the floor to a count of two).

Too easy? Cross your arms on your chest.

8 STRENGTHENING: Quadruped single leg lift

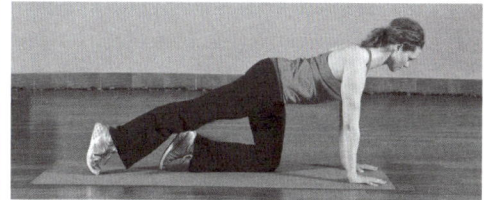
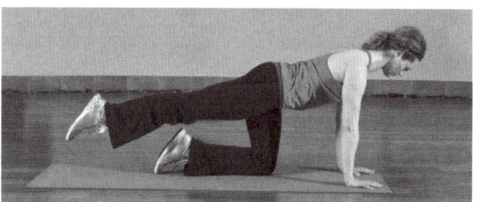

Reps: 10 on each side **Sets:** 1–3 **Intensity:** Light to moderate
Tempo: 3-1-3 **Rest:** 30–90 seconds between sets

Starting position: Position yourself on hands and knees ("all fours") on the floor.

Movement: Extend your right leg behind you, slowly lifting it up to hip level. Pause, then return to the starting position. Finish all reps, then repeat with your left leg. This completes one set.

Tips and techniques:
- Keep your shoulders and hips even.
- Maintain a neutral spine.
- Contract your abdominal muscles throughout.

Too hard? Lie on your stomach, resting your chin on your hands. Slowly lift one leg off the floor. Pause, then slowly return to the starting position. Finish all reps, then repeat with the opposite leg.

Too easy? Add 1- to 3-pound ankle weights.

9 STRETCHING: Kneeling hip flexor stretch

Reps: 3–4 **Sets:** 1 **Intensity:** Moderate
Hold: 10–30 seconds **Rest:** No rest needed

Starting position: Kneel on the mat.
Movement: Put your right leg in front of you with the knee bent at a 90-degree angle and foot flat on the floor. You may place your hands on your right thigh for support. Lean forward, pressing into the hip of your left leg while keeping your right foot on the floor. Hold. Finish all reps, then switch legs. This completes one set.

Tips and techniques:
- Stretch to the point of mild tension, not pain.
- Maintain a neutral spine while keeping hips and shoulders even.
- Keep your shoulders down and back, and your abdominal muscles contracted.

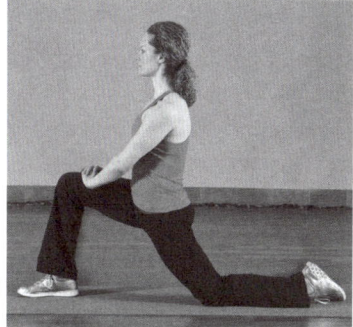

Too hard? Lie on your back. Pull your right knee toward your chest and extend your left leg on the floor. Flex your left foot and press your left calf down into the floor. You'll feel this stretch at the front of the extended leg, the lower back, and the buttock of the bent knee. Hold. Finish all reps, then switch legs to repeat.

Too easy? As you lean forward, pressing into the hip of your left leg, lift your left arm up and over as if raising your hand in class.

www.health.harvard.edu   The Joint Pain Relief Workout   33

HIP WORKOUT

10 STRETCHING: Gluteal stretch

Reps: 3–4
Sets: 1
Intensity: Moderate
Hold: 10–30 seconds
Rest: No rest needed

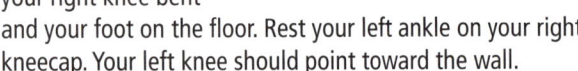

Starting position: Lie on your back with your right knee bent and your foot on the floor. Rest your left ankle on your right kneecap. Your left knee should point toward the wall.

Movement: Hold the back of the right thigh with both hands and slowly lift your right foot up off the floor until you feel the stretch in your left hip and buttock. Hold. Return to the starting position, then repeat on the opposite side. This is one rep. Continue alternating leg positions until you finish all reps.

Tips and techniques:
- Stretch to the point of mild tension, not pain.
- Relax your shoulders down and back into the floor.
- Breathe comfortably.

Too hard? Lie on your back with both knees bent and your feet flat on the floor. Cross your right knee over your left knee and pull your knees in toward your chest. Repeat with your left knee crossed over your right knee. This is one rep.

Too easy? Lie on your back with your right knee bent and your foot on the floor. Rest your left ankle on your right kneecap. Clasp your right knee with both hands and lift your right foot up off the floor. Repeat with your right ankle on your left kneecap. This is one rep.

11 STRETCHING: Cobbler's pose

Reps: 3–4
Sets: 1
Intensity: Moderate
Hold: 10–30 seconds
Rest: No rest needed

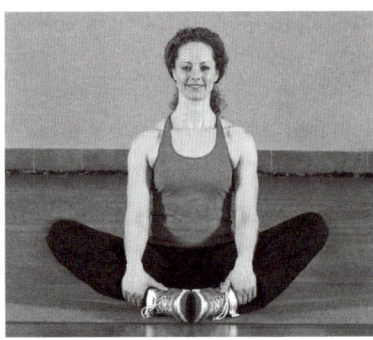

Starting position: Sit on the floor. Bring the soles of your feet together and let your knees fall apart toward the floor.

Movement: Place your hands on your ankles. Hinge forward from your hips until you feel the stretch in your inner thighs. Hold.

Tips and techniques:
- Stretch to the point of mild tension, not pain.
- Maintain a neutral head and spine with your shoulders down and back and abdominal muscles contracted.
- Breathe comfortably.

Too hard? Perform the cobbler's stretch while lying on your back.

Too easy? Sit against a wall and pull in your feet for a greater stretch.

12 STRETCHING: Hamstring stretch

Reps: 3–4   **Sets:** 1   **Intensity:** Moderate
Hold: 10–30 seconds   **Rest:** No rest needed

Starting position: Lie on your back with both knees bent and feet flat on the floor.

Movement: Hold your right leg with both hands behind the thigh. Lift your right foot toward the ceiling as you extend your knee. Straighten the leg as much as possible without locking the knee. As you do so, flex the ankle to stretch the calf muscles. Hold. Repeat with the left leg. This is one rep. Continue alternating leg positions until you finish all reps.

Tips and techniques:
- Stretch the leg extended toward the ceiling to the point of mild tension without any pressure behind the knee or any pain.
- Relax your shoulders down and back into the floor.
- Breathe comfortably.

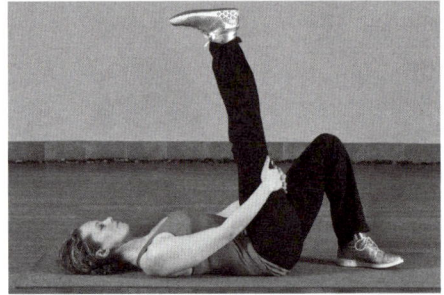

Too hard? Sit up straight in a chair and extend one leg straight out in front of you with the toes pointing to the ceiling. Hinge forward from the hip while maintaining a neutral spine. Finish all reps, then repeat with other leg.

Too easy? Stand upright and extend one leg straight in front of you with your foot on a chair or counter. Flex your ankle. Hinge forward from the hip while maintaining a neutral spine. Finish all reps, then repeat with other leg.

Shoulder workout

While busy hands often get all the credit, the most mundane daily tasks—brushing your hair, sweeping your wallet off the dresser, reaching for the front doorknob—can't be done unless your shoulders position your arms and hands in the right spots.

Shoulders 101

Although we refer to the shoulder as if it were a single joint, in reality four joints loosely connect several bones. Riding above the rib cage are four bones that form the shoulder girdle: a pair of collarbones (clavicles) at the front, and a pair of triangular shoulder blades or wing bones (scapulae) at the back. The inner end of each collarbone is linked to the breastbone (sternum). The outer end of the collarbone fits into a small joint meeting up with the front edge of the shoulder blade (forming the acromioclavicular, or AC, joint), so that the four bones largely float above the ribs, suspended by several strong muscles and ligaments.

The long bone of the upper arm (humerus) fits into a larger ball-and-socket joint at the shoulder blade (see Figure 5). This allows the arm to move freely in many directions, making it possible to serve a tennis ball or push a vacuum. Yet it also makes the shoulder joint inherently unstable and easy to injure.

A tendon bridging four small muscles creates the rotator cuff. The cuff covers the ball of the shoulder joint and permits you to rotate your arm and stabilizes the joint. Even a basic action, like lifting your arm, requires every part of the shoulder girdle to move in turn and calls into play rotator cuff muscles plus a raft of strong muscles of the shoulders, back, and chest.

What this workout helps

- **Shoulder impingement.** A common cause of shoulder pain occurs when the front portion of the shoulder blade impinges on the rotator cuff as you raise your arm. This may cause bursitis or tendinitis or a tear in the rotator cuff. Shoulder impingement causes pain and limits movement considerably, occasionally creating a "frozen shoulder." Common causes include overuse of rotator cuff muscles in sports like tennis, swimming, and baseball, work like painting that repeatedly involves reaching overhead, and minor injuries.

- **Osteoarthritis.** Sometimes dubbed "wear and tear" arthritis because it starts when cartilage cushioning the joints wears down, osteoarthritis of the shoulder is a common cause of pain in people over age 50. Prior injuries, aging, and overuse are all factors.

- **Bursitis.** Small, fluid-filled sacs called bursae cushion the movement of bones against muscle, skin, and tendons. Bursae above the rotator cuff are prime candidates for inflammation (bursitis) prompted by causes similar to those for shoulder impingement or because of anatomical factors.

- **Tendinitis.** Shoulder impingement may lead to pain, swelling, and inflammation of the rotator cuff tendon.

Figure 5 Anatomy of the shoulder joint

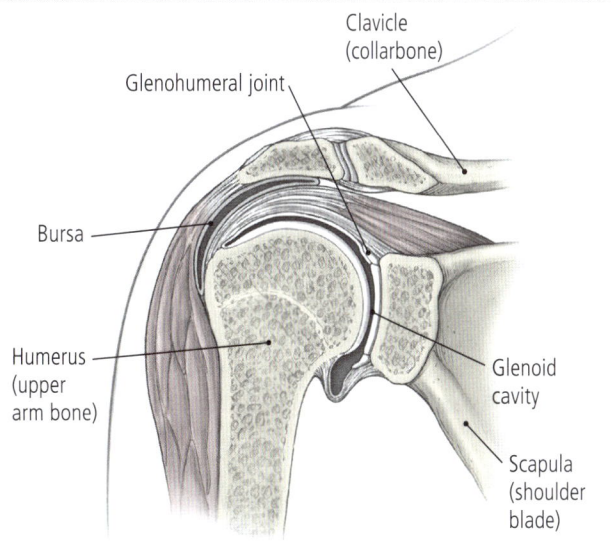

Many shoulder injuries involve the shoulder's main joint, where the humerus connects with the shoulder socket (called the glenoid) at the scapula.

SHOULDER WORKOUT

Shoulder exercises

As the least stable joint in your body, your shoulders will benefit from exercises designed to strengthen supporting muscles while gently increasing your range of motion, so that you can easily swing a golf club or reach overhead, for example. Impingements that prevent movements like these are often a result of poor shoulder flexibility and impaired movement patterns. Maintaining strength and flexibility in your shoulder also reduces stress across the joint, making you less susceptible to bursitis and tendinitis.

For the first two weeks: Do only the warm-ups and stretches. Practice at least two to three times a week or as often as daily.

Starting at week 3: Begin to perform the full workout two to three times a week. Make sure you leave 48 hours between strength exercise sessions to allow muscles time to recover. Warm-ups and stretches can be done daily to further enhance flexibility.

Equipment: 1- to 3-pound hand weights, resistance tubing with door attachment, stability ball, hand towel.

1 WARMING UP: Shoulder circles

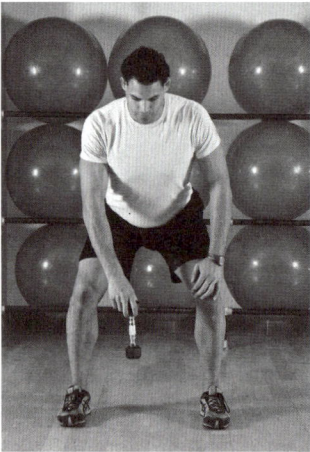

Reps: 20 per arm
Sets: 1
Intensity: Light
Tempo: Slow and controlled
Rest: No rest needed

Starting position: Stand up straight with your feet hip-width apart. Hold a 1- to 3-pound weight in your right hand with one end of the weight hanging down toward the floor.

Movement: Bend your knees a bit and slightly hinge forward from the hip so that you're holding the weight between your legs. You can rest your left hand on your left thigh for support. Make 10 circles in one direction with your right arm as if stirring a pot. Pause, then reverse direction for 10 circles. Repeat with your left arm (again performing both clockwise and counter-clockwise circles). This completes one set.

Tips and techniques:
- Hinge from the hips without bending or arching your back.
- Maintain neutral posture with your shoulders down and back.
- Allow the weight to hang like a dead weight.

Too hard? Perform the exercise while seated, or try it standing with no weight.
Too easy? Make a larger circle.

2 WARMING UP: Shoulder pendulums

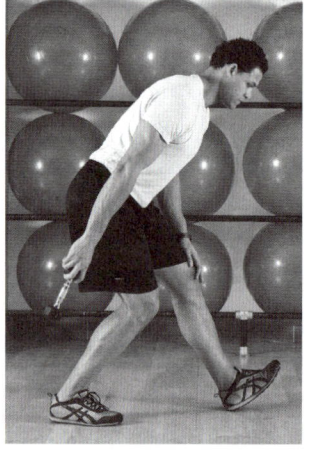 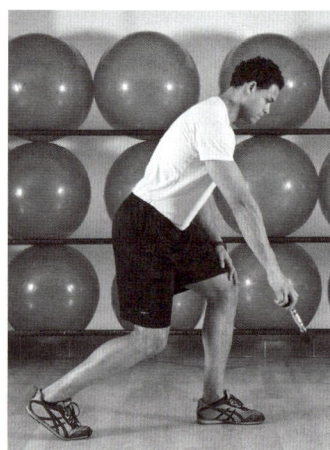

Reps: 10 **Sets:** 1 **Intensity:** Light
Tempo: Slow and controlled
Rest: No rest needed

Starting position: Stand up straight with your feet together. Hold a 1- to 3-pound weight in your right hand with one end of the weight hanging down toward the floor.

Movement: Extend your right leg straight back and press the right heel toward the floor, bending your left knee slightly. Slowly rock your body forward and back, allowing the weight to swing gently like a pendulum. Finish all reps, then switch positions and repeat with the weight in your left hand.

Tips and techniques:
- Maintain neutral posture with your shoulders down and back.
- Slant your whole body forward by hinging from the ankles.
- Rock back and forth, lifting the heel of the back leg and then the toe of the front leg.

Too hard? Perform the exercise while seated, or try it standing with no weight.
Too easy? Make a larger arc as you swing the weight like a pendulum.

SHOULDER WORKOUT

3 STRENGTHENING: Wall push-up with stability ball

Reps: 10 **Sets:** 1–3
Intensity: Moderate **Tempo:** 3-1-3
Rest: 30–90 seconds between sets

Starting position: Facing a wall, stand up straight to position a stability ball against the wall at shoulder height. Your arms should be extended at chest height with your palms against the ball, fingertips pointing toward the ceiling.

Movement: Slowly bend your elbows to lower your upper body toward the ball, keeping a straight line from head to heel. Pause, then slowly push away from the ball to return to the starting position. Throughout the movement, maintain neutral alignment from head to toe.

Tips and techniques:
- Keep your fingertips no higher than shoulder level.
- Keep your elbows close to your sides as you bend them.
- Keep your shoulders down and back.

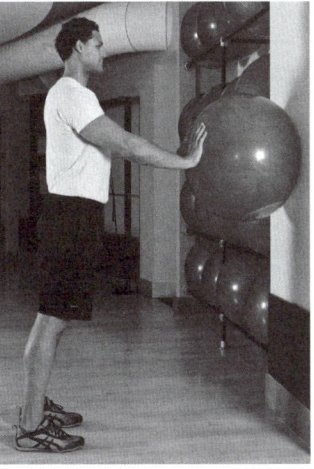 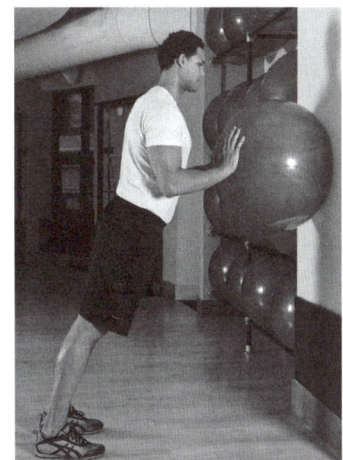

Too hard? Try the wall push-up without the stability ball.
Too easy? After you lower your body toward the ball, hold the position for a count of eight. Then slowly push away from the ball to return to the starting position.

4 STRENGTHENING: Standing internal and external rotation

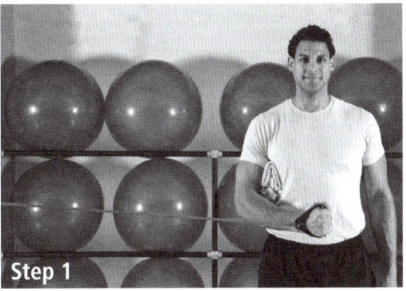
Step 1

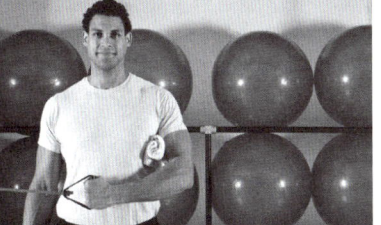
Step 2a

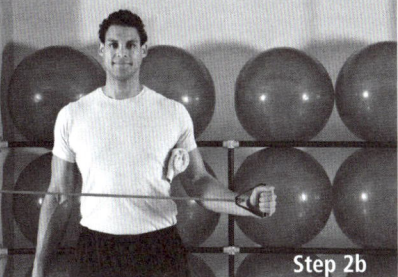
Step 2b

Reps: 10 **Sets:** 1–3
Intensity: Moderate to hard
Tempo: 3-1-3
Rest: 30–90 seconds between sets

Starting position: Anchor the resistance tubing to a door at waist level. Stand with your feet hip-width apart. Grasp one handle of the tubing in your right hand with your thumb pointed at the ceiling and your elbow firmly pinning a hand towel at your side. Turn your body so that your right side faces the door, keeping tension on the tubing throughout the exercise.

Movement: This is a two-step exercise. *Step 1:* Keep your wrist firm as you slowly pull the band in toward your bellybutton like a door closing. Pause, then slowly return to the starting position. Finish all reps.
Step 2: Switch hands so that you are grasping the handle with your left hand across your waist, knuckles near your bellybutton, and your left elbow pinning the hand towel at your side. (If necessary, adjust the tension on the resistance tubing by moving a bit closer to or farther away from the door.) Keep your wrist firm as you slowly pull the tubing outward like a door opening. Pause, then slowly return to the starting position. Finish all reps. Turn your body so that your left side faces the door and repeat both steps. This completes one set.

Tips and techniques:
- Maintain neutral posture with your shoulders down and back.
- Maintain a firm, neutral wrist.
- Keep the hand towel under your working elbow as an anchor point.

Too hard? Use lighter resistance tubing.
Too easy? Use heavier resistance tubing.

SHOULDER WORKOUT

5 STRENGTHENING: Standing V-raise

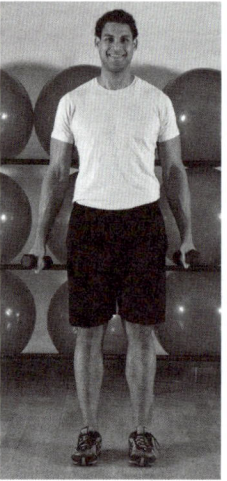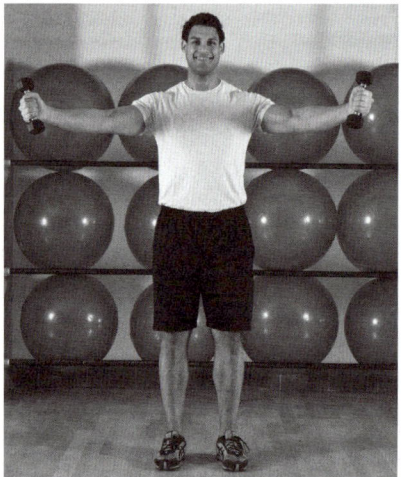

Reps: 10   **Sets:** 1–3   **Intensity:** Moderate
Tempo: 3-1-3   **Rest:** 30–90 seconds between sets

Starting position: Stand up straight holding 1- to 3-pound weights with your hands at your sides, thumbs facing forward. Position your feet hip-width apart.

Movement: Squeeze your shoulder blades together while you slowly lift your arms, creating a V as you raise the weights. Go no higher than your shoulders. Pause, then slowly return to the starting position.

Tips and techniques:
- Keep your wrists firm, maintaining a straight line from your elbow to your knuckles, and elbows soft (not locked) throughout the movement.
- Maintain neutral posture with your shoulders down and back.
- Exhale as you lift.

Too hard? Use a lighter weight.
Too easy? Use a heavier weight.

6 STRENGTHENING: Standing row

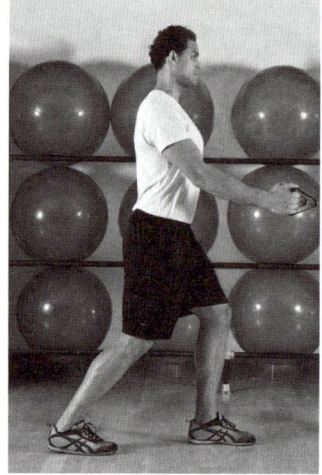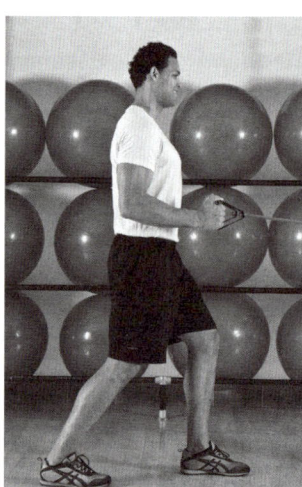

Reps: 10   **Sets:** 1–3   **Intensity:** Moderate
Tempo: 3-1-3   **Rest:** 30–90 seconds between sets

Starting position: Anchor the resistance tubing to a door at chest height. Stand up straight facing the door with your feet together. Stand far enough away from the door to put tension on the tubing as you hold the handles with your arms extended. Extend your right leg straight back and press the right heel toward the floor, bending both knees slightly.

Movement: Squeeze your shoulder blades together. Slowly bend your arms and pull back. Keep your elbows close to your ribs and pointing toward the back wall. Pause, then slowly return to the starting position.

Tips and techniques:
- Maintain neutral posture with your shoulders down and back and your wrists firm.
- Exhale as you pull.

Too hard? Use lighter resistance tubing.
Too easy? Use heavier resistance tubing.

7 STRENGTHENING: Biceps curl

Reps: 10   **Sets:** 1–3   **Intensity:** Light to moderate
Tempo: 3-1-3   **Rest:** 30–90 seconds between sets

Starting position: Stand up straight with your feet hip-width apart, holding 1- to 3-pound weights at your side with your palms facing forward.

Movement: Slowly bend your elbows to lift the weights up to the front of your shoulders. Exhale as you lift. Pause. Slowly lower them to the starting position.

Tips and techniques:
- Keep your shoulders still, down, and back.
- Keep your wrists neutral and your elbows stationary at the sides of your ribs throughout the movement.

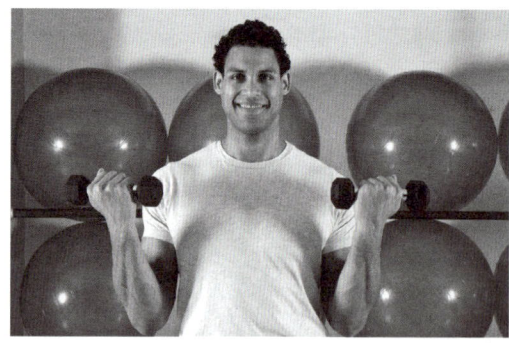

Too hard? Use lighter weights.
Too easy? Use heavier weights.

The Joint Pain Relief Workout

SHOULDER WORKOUT

8 STRENGTHENING: Diagonals

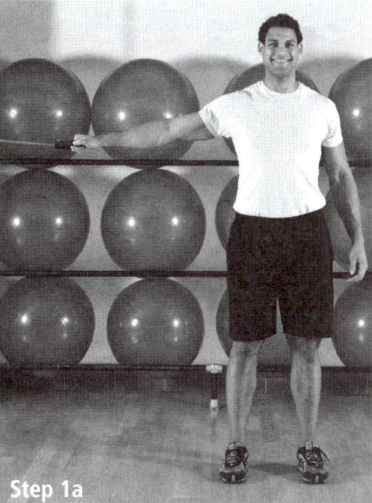
Step 1a

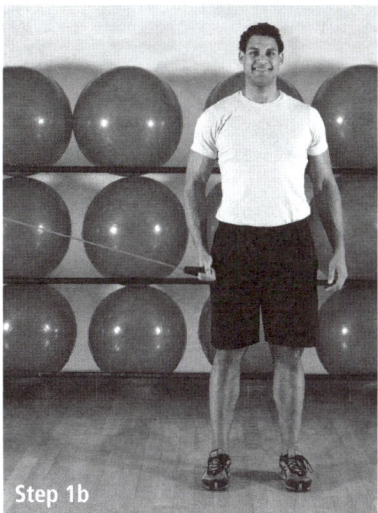
Step 1b

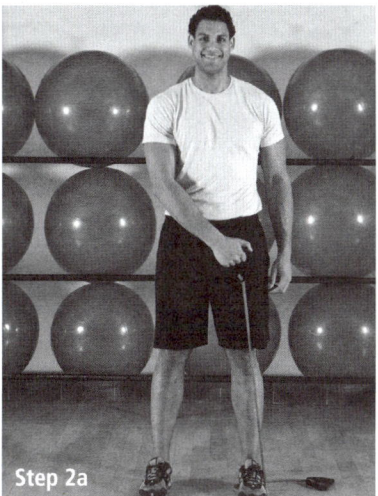
Step 2a

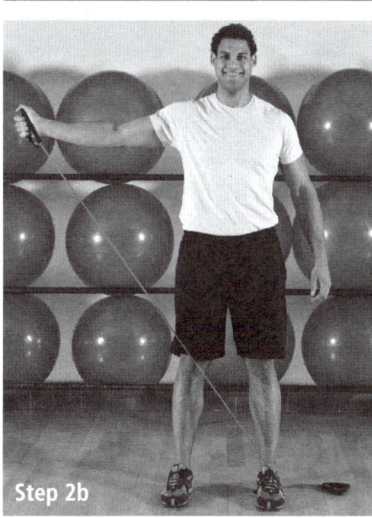
Step 2b

Reps: 10
Sets: 1–3
Intensity: Moderate
Tempo: 3-1-3
Rest: 30–90 seconds between sets

Starting position: Anchor resistance tubing to a door at chest level. Stand with your right side to the door. Position your legs hip-width apart, chest up, and shoulders down and back. Grasp the handle of the tubing in your right hand with your arm held out straight just below shoulder height, thumb facing forward. Keep tension on the tubing throughout the exercise.

Movement: This is a two-step exercise.
Step 1: Keeping your wrist firm and arm straight, slowly pull your right arm down toward your right hip. Pause, then slowly return to the starting position. Finish all reps, then stand with your left side to the door and repeat, grasping the handle in your left hand.
Step 2: Anchor the resistance tubing to the floor with your left foot. Hold the handle with your right hand near your left hip, thumb toward the wall. Keeping your wrist firm, slowly lift your right hand up on a diagonal to shoulder height. Pause, then slowly bring your right hand back to your left hip. Finish all reps with the right arm before anchoring the tubing under your right foot and repeating with your left arm. This completes one set.

Tips and techniques:
- You may need to use lighter resistance tubing on this exercise to complete the movement with good form and ease.
- Keep your wrist firm and your shoulders down and back.
- Exhale as you pull.

Too hard? Use lighter resistance tubing.
Too easy? Use heavier resistance tubing.

SHOULDER WORKOUT

9 STRETCHING: Shoulder stretch

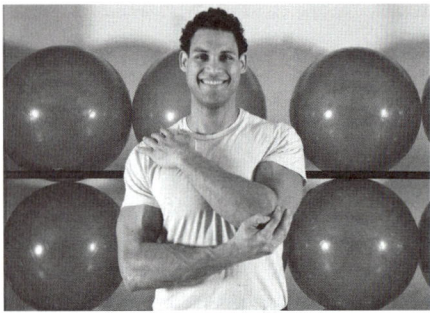

Reps: 3–4
Sets: 1
Intensity: Light
Hold: 10–30 seconds
Rest: No rest needed

Starting position: Stand with your feet hip-width apart. Put your left hand on your right shoulder. Cup your left elbow with your right hand.

Movement: Roll your shoulders down and back as you gently pull your left elbow across your chest. Hold. Return to the starting position. Finish all reps, then repeat on the other side.

Tips and techniques:
- Stretch to the point of mild tension, not pain.
- Keep your shoulders down and back.
- Breathe comfortably.

Too hard? Stretch only as far as is comfortable.
Too easy? Repeat the stretch several times during the day.

10 STRETCHING: Wall climb

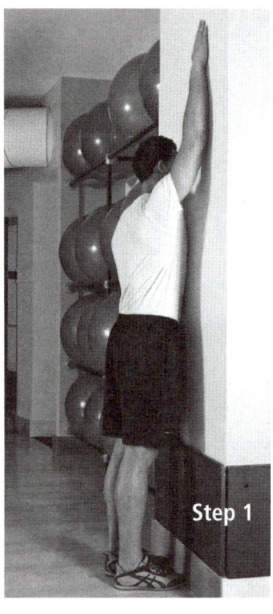
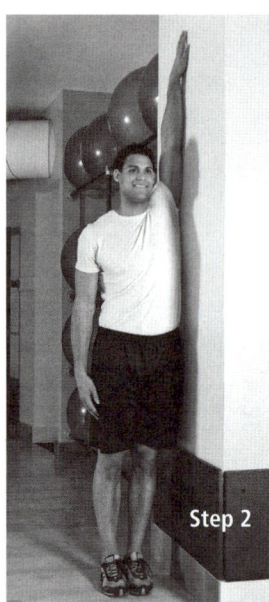

Step 1   Step 2

Reps: 3–4
Sets: 1
Intensity: Light to moderate
Hold: 10–30 seconds
Rest: No rest needed

Starting position: Stand up straight facing a wall.

Movement: This is a two-part exercise. *Step 1:* Extend your right arm with your elbow soft (not locked) and place your hand on the wall at shoulder height. Slowly walk your fingers upward, stepping in toward the wall as your hand climbs higher. Stop when you feel mild tension. Hold. Slowly walk your fingers back down the wall and return to the starting position. Finish all reps. *Step 2:* Turn so that your right side faces the wall. Extend your right arm with your elbow soft (not locked) and place your hand on the wall at shoulder height. Slowly walk your fingers upward, stepping in toward the wall as your hand climbs higher. Stop when you feel mild tension. Hold. Slowly walk your fingers back down the wall and return to the starting position. Finish all reps. Repeat both steps using your left hand. This completes the set.

Tips and techniques:
- Stretch to the point of mild tension, not pain.
- Progress slowly toward the goal of bringing your body right next to the wall.
- Breathe comfortably.

Too hard? Place your hand on the wall below shoulder height and go only as high as is comfortable.
Too easy? Repeat the stretch several times throughout the day.

SHOULDER WORKOUT

11 STRETCHING: Shoulder stretch with internal rotation

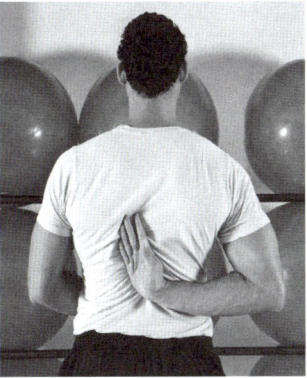

Reps: 3–4 **Sets:** 1
Intensity: Moderate
Hold: 10–30 seconds
Rest: No rest needed

Starting position: Stand up straight with your feet hip-width apart and your hands by your sides.

Movement: Place the back of your right hand against the small of your back at your waist. Your thumb should be pointing up. Slowly slide your right hand farther up your back as high as you can. Hold. Finish all reps, then repeat with your left hand.

Tips and techniques:
- Stretch to the point of mild tension, not pain.
- Maintain neutral posture with your shoulders down and back.
- Breathe comfortably.

Too hard? Make your movement smaller.

Too easy? Repeat the stretch several times during the day.

12 STRETCHING: Chest stretch

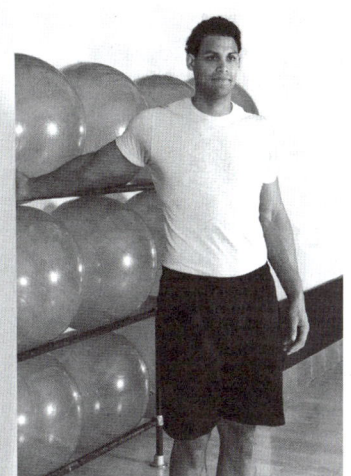

Reps: 3–4
Sets: 1
Intensity: Light to moderate
Hold: 10–30 seconds
Rest: No rest needed

Starting position: Stand in a doorway facing forward. Extend your right arm and put your right hand on the edge of the doorframe slightly below shoulder level, palm facing forward and touching the doorframe. Keep your shoulders down and back.

Movement: Slowly turn your body to the left, away from the doorframe, until you feel the stretch in your chest and shoulder. Hold. Return to the starting position. Finish all reps, then repeat on the opposite side.

Tips and techniques:
- Stretch to the point of mild tension, not pain.
- Breathe comfortably.

Too hard? Put your hand a bit lower on the doorframe and don't turn as far.

Too easy? Repeat the stretch several times during the day.

Wrist and elbow mini-workout

If you're an avid athlete sidelined by tennis elbow or golfer's elbow, or an office athlete wincing from job-related repetitive motions, this workout can get you back in the game by enhancing flexibility and strengthening supporting muscles. We recommend performing the full workout two to three times a week.

One additional easy exercise—squeezing a rubber ball 30 times at a slow, controlled pace—needs no illustration and can be practiced daily to improve your grip. The squishier the ball, the easier the workout, so choose a firmer rubber ball when you're ready for more of a challenge. If you have arthritis, try putting your hands in warm water while squeezing the ball.

Equipment: Hand weights (1 to 3 pounds), sturdy chair, rubber ball.

WARMING UP AND STRETCHING

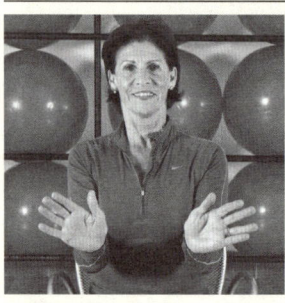 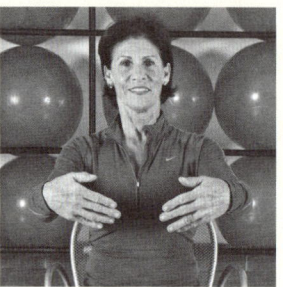 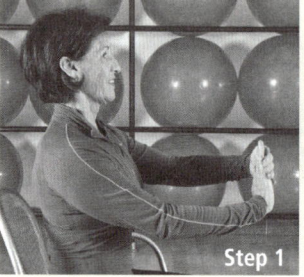 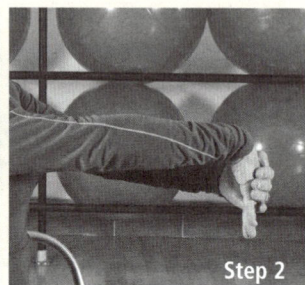

Step 1   Step 2

1. Wrist circle warm-up

Reps: 10
Sets: 1–3
Intensity: Light
Tempo: Slow and controlled
Rest: No rest needed

Starting position: Sit in a chair or stand up straight.
Movement: Slowly circle your wrists 10 times in one direction and 10 times in the other direction. This is one complete set.

Tips and techniques:
- Maintain neutral posture with your shoulders down and back.
- Breathe comfortably.

> **Too hard?** Make smaller circles.
> **Too easy?** Repeat the warm-up several times throughout the day.

2. Wrist stretch

Reps: 3–4
Sets: 1
Intensity: Light
Hold: 10–30 seconds
Rest: No rest needed

Starting position: Sit in a chair with your right arm and hand extended in front of you with the palm down, facing the floor.
Movement: This is a two-step exercise. *Step one:* Point the fingers of your right hand toward the ceiling. Place the palm of your left hand in front of your right hand to extend your wrist. Gently press your left hand against the palm and fingers of your right hand to increase the stretch, stopping if you feel any pain. Hold. Return to the starting position. *Step two:* Bend your right hand forward at the wrist, pointing your fingers downward into a fully flexed position. Cup the back of your right hand with your left hand. Gently press downward with your left hand to increase the stretch, stopping if you feel any pain. Hold. Finish all reps, then switch arms and repeat both steps on your left hand.

Tips and techniques:
- Stretch to the point of mild tension, not pain.
- Maintain neutral posture with your shoulders down and back.
- Breathe comfortably.

> **Too hard?** Press more gently to limit the range of motion.
> **Too easy?** Repeat the stretch several times throughout the day.

STRENGTHENING

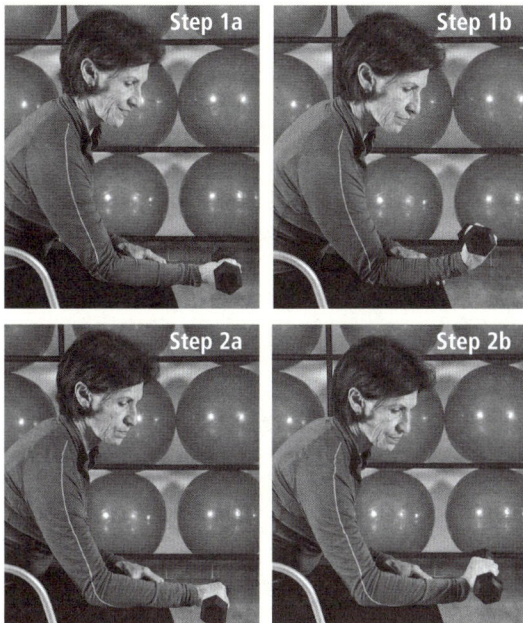

3. Wrist flexion and extension

Reps: 10
Sets: 1–3
Intensity: Light
Tempo: 3-1-3
Rest: 30–90 seconds between sets

Starting position: Sit in a chair holding a 1-pound weight in your right hand, palm facing up and wrist neutral. Lean forward, bending at the hip, and place the back of your right forearm on your thigh.

Movement: This is a two-step exercise. *Step 1:* Slowly curl your right hand upward. Pause, then slowly return to the starting position so that your wrist is neutral. Finish all reps, then repeat with your left hand holding the weight. *Step 2:* Reverse the exercise. Hold the light weight in your right hand, palm facing down, wrist neutral, and forearm supported on your thigh. Slowly bend your wrist backward to lift up the weight. Pause, and slowly return to the neutral wrist position. Finish all reps, then repeat with your left hand holding the weight. This completes one set.

Tips and techniques:
- Maintain neutral posture with your shoulders down and back.
- Be sure to return to a neutral wrist at the beginning and end of each rep.
- Breathe comfortably, exhaling as you lift.

Too hard? Use a lighter weight or no weight.
Too easy? Use a heavier weight.

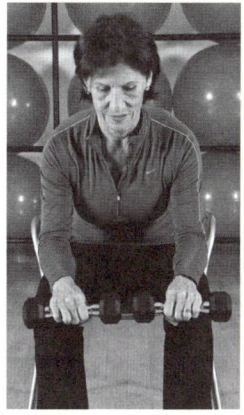 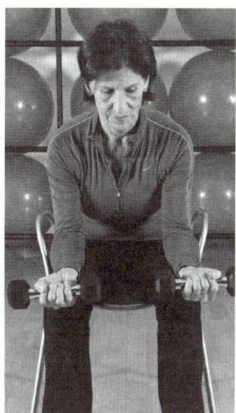

4. Palm up, palm down

Reps: 10
Sets: 1–3
Intensity: Light
Tempo: 3-1-3
Rest: 30–90 seconds between sets

Starting position: Sit in a chair holding a 1-pound weight in each hand with your elbows slightly bent and your palms facing the floor. Your wrists should be neutral.

Movement: Slowly turn your hands over until your palms face the ceiling. Pause, then slowly return to the starting position.

Tips and techniques:
- Maintain neutral posture with your shoulders down and back.
- Keep your wrists neutral throughout the movement.
- Breathe comfortably.

Too hard? Use lighter weights or no weights.
Too easy? Use heavier weights.

Resources

Publications

The No Sweat Exercise Plan
Harvey B. Simon, M.D.
(McGraw-Hill, 2006)

A founding member of the Harvard Cardiovascular Health Center, Dr. Simon sets forth an engaging no-sweat exercise plan based upon solid research. An easy-to-follow point system helps readers tailor fitness programs to their own needs and measure health benefits from everyday activities and numerous sports.

Exercise: A Program You Can Live With
L. Howard Hartley, M.D., and I-Min Lee, M.B., B.S., Sc.D.
(Harvard Medical School, 2012)

A guide to starting and maintaining an exercise program that suits your abilities and lifestyle. This Special Health Report from Harvard Medical School also offers advice on fitness products.

Walk with Ease
Arthritis Foundation, 3rd Edition
(Arthritis Foundation, 2009)

An easy-to-follow walking program designed for people with arthritis. The program is intended to be adapted depending on needs, which are determined through self-assessments. Includes information on different types of arthritis, why certain activities are especially helpful, what to do if exercise hurts, and positive solutions for problems that could crop up.

Workout Workbook: 9 Complete Workouts to Help You Get Fit and Healthy
Jonathan F. Bean, M.D., M.S., M.P.H., along with personal trainers Joy Prouty and Josie Gardiner
(Harvard Medical School, 2009)

This Special Health Report from Harvard Medical School includes nine excellent workouts to try at home, take on the road, or mix into your gym routine. Core, strength, stability ball, power challenge, travel, and other workouts help you bump up activity and enhance fitness. Also includes warm-up and cool-down routines.

Organizations

American Academy of Physical Medicine and Rehabilitation
9700 W. Bryn Mawr Ave., Suite 200
Rosemont, IL 60018
847-737-6000

A national professional organization for physiatrists—medical doctors trained in physical medicine and rehabilitation—which promotes education and funds research in this area. A referral service on the website locates physiatrists state-by-state.

American College of Sports Medicine
401 W. Michigan St.
Indianapolis, IN 46202
317-637-9200

ACSM educates and certifies fitness professionals, such as personal trainers, and funds research on exercise. A referral service on the website locates ASCM-certified personal trainers.

American Council on Exercise
4851 Paramount Drive
San Diego, CA 92123
888-825-3636 (toll-free)

ACE is a nonprofit organization that promotes fitness and offers a wide array of educational materials for consumers and professionals. Their website offers a library of free exercise videos and a referral service to locate ACE-certified personal trainers.

American Physical Therapy Association
1111 N. Fairfax St.
Alexandria, VA 22314
800-999-2782 (toll-free)

This national professional organization fosters advances in physical therapy education, research, and practice. A referral system on the website locates board-certified clinical specialists with additional training in specific areas.

Arthritis Foundation
P.O. Box 7669
Atlanta, GA 30357
800-283-7800 (toll-free)

A national not-for-profit organization with local chapters in many states. The website offers educational materials on arthritis, pain control, treatments, alternative therapies, and more, as well as exercise videos. Local chapters may offer classes, such as Walk with Ease, a six-week, instructor-led walking program designed for people with arthritis.

National Institute on Aging (NIA)
Building 31, Room 5C27
31 Center Drive, MSC 2292
Bethesda, MD 20892
301-496-1752
www.nia.nih.gov/Go4Life

Part of the National Institutes of Health, the National Institute on Aging has a free, easy-to-follow booklet and companion video packed with good exercises called *Exercise & Physical Activity*. These can be viewed online or ordered by phone. The NIA's Go4Life website hosts an exercise and activity campaign aimed at enhancing endurance, strength, balance, and flexibility for people ages 50 and older, including those recovering from injuries or living with chronic illnesses.

Weight-Control Information Network
1 WIN Way
Bethesda, MD 20892
877-946-4627 (toll-free)

This government service, part of the National Institutes of Health, offers free publications on obesity, weight control, and nutrition.